Talking
About Walking the Dog

Journeying Towards Self-Compassion with ADHD

Katy Fraser

Talking to a Pie About Walking the Dog
By Katy Fraser

© Katy Fraser

ISBN: 978-1-911740-15-5

First published in 2025

Managing editor: Bridget Reaume
Proofreader: Andreea Marina Grijincu
Cover Design: Tasmin Briers

Published by Palavro, an imprint of
the Arkbound Foundation (Publishers)

Arkbound is a social enterprise that aims to promote social
inclusion, community development and artistic talent. It
sponsors publications by disadvantaged authors and covers
issues that engage wider social concerns. Arkbound fully
embraces sustainability and environmental protection. It
endeavours to use material that is renewable, recyclable or
sourced from sustainable forest.

Arkbound
1-3, Gloucester Rd,
Bishopston, Bristol BS7 8AA

www.arkbound.com

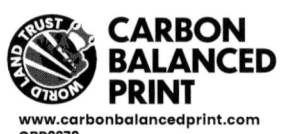

www.carbonbalancedprint.com
CBP2278

Talking to a Pie About Walking the Dog

Journeying Towards Self-Compassion with ADHD

Katy Fraser

Supporters

The publication of this book was enabled through a dedicated crowdfunding campaign on Crowdbound.org.

Among the many supporters, we are particularly grateful to:

Martin Walker
Margareta Allison
Diana Forsythe
Stacie Standing
Yasmin Clarke
Saba Alai
Grant Otto
Joseph Fletcher
Nicole Yip
Sinead Myerscough
Matthew Azoulay
Ruby Clachan
Aurelie Proisy
Frida Burnet
Tommy Standing
Danny Standing
Sandra Carberry

Contents

Part Two:
The Huge Wordless Question

Part Three:
Talking to a Pie About Walking the Dog

For my grandchildren.

Introduction

'If you are always trying to be normal,
you will never know how amazing
you can be.' – Maya Angelou.

This is not a book about getting things done. It is written to and for the innermost essence of people with ADHD neurology. It's not about just productivity, spontaneity, or chaos versus calm; this is a book about us. Our 'beingness.'

When – for years or decades – we have felt at odds with the world and then we learn we have ADHD neurology, in the light of our new understanding, we might begin to gently reframe our experiences. To look at ourselves through kinder eyes. Kindness we so quickly offer to others in times of difficulty and so rarely extend to ourselves.

For those of us who did not discover our puzzle's 'missing pieces' until adulthood, this book is for you! This book is a journey towards discovering new self-identities, confidence, and compassion.

Following a diagnosis, we might feel angry or sad about having been misunderstood, and unsure of how to move forward. So, finding ways to make peace with past confusions and establishing a loving place for ourselves matters.

Refocusing our scope to a kinder lens can also help us make sense of our lives and self-view before diagnosis. I have written this book as a self-compassion exercise, and it has been uncomfortable to acknowledge how unkind my self-view was.

Now, in collaboration with neurodivergent people, I have observed firsthand that when families, schools, universities, or workplaces aren't 'up to speed' about neurodiversity, there is much (often quiet and unnoticed) suffering. It matters to work authentically with my clients and guide them toward finding kinder ways to speak and look at themselves until the world 'catches up.'

The anecdotes in this book offer examples of the typically confusing experiences about selfhood that someone with undiagnosed ADHD or AuDHD might have.

In this book, the terms are used

interchangeably. At the time of writing, AuDHD is a colloquial term describing people with two types of neurodivergence – but it does not exist as an official diagnosis in the Diagnostic and Statistical Manual-5 (DSM-5). (Watch this space!)

AuDHD is becoming a widely recognized term describing people with two types of neurodivergence: Autism and Attention Deficit Hyperactivity Disorder. Studies indicate that fifty percent of people with Autism also have ADHD. The experience of AuDHD might be described as a complementary clash between traits, as aspects of each neurotype often overlap. While these traits can blend and interact beautifully, it's not unusual to feel confused or contradictory until the possibility of AuDHD is on our radar. When we begin to explore how these complements and clashes show up in our lives, self-compassion becomes a tool to remind us that these are aspects of our humanness—not definitions of who we are.

Like me, you may have received your diagnosis with relief, alarm, or a mixture of those feelings. Finally understanding what is 'going on' can be at odds with how we view ourselves. In some ways, diagnosis is just the beginning of our journey!

Through everyday tales of being in the world, I hope to illustrate that the journey toward self-compassion with ADHD can be exciting and worthwhile. I will invite you alongside me, Dear Reader, to view neurodiversity through a compassionate lens. I am already grateful for your company.

Prologue
The Abstract Wonder that is ADHD

'Humans struggle with the underside of the tapestry, unable to see the beauty in their situation, for they cannot know how the trouble of life fits with The Plan' – Chris Fabry.

Depicted in a tapestry, our lives as people with ADHD might offer a definable picture. There may be some noticeable wrong stitches, patching over; nevertheless, it's likely a colourful work. There may be texture in places – fuzzy, like homespun wool – with brightness nestled within, giving the piece the kind of difference that makes its viewer startle slightly.

Diagnosed with ADHD in my early fifties, it was time to fathom my tapestry. The front was a discernible picture but flipping it over revealed – unsurprisingly – an elaborate mess. One that looked exactly like how living life felt.

This tapestry might belong to any

neurodivergent adult. As I did, you may recognise your knotting as confusion and the long back-threading to be your mighty efforts, which appear in those few brief-but-bright stitches on the front.

To heal the disharmony between my life's picture and the truth of my experience has meant embracing the whole work. It's been both bewildering and relieving to realise that many of the fibres I always sought to extract were integral to the thread itself.

So, if you happen to find yourself here, Dear Reader, it is my sincere hope that it might bring you to consider the threads of your own tapestry – where your unique experience of neurodiversity lies flat, knots, puckers and shines.

As long as it's still being stitched and its fibres are handled with care, the threads of our unique story can stitch countless shapes and allow our struggles to reframe as possibilities.

Part One:

It's Not about Socks

The Right Questions

'Asking the right questions takes as much skill as giving the right answers.' – Robert Half.

1970

Once, there was a little girl who knew her wholeness. Under the sky, among the flowers, there was no reason to make up for something she felt was lacking. Yet, somehow, as she moved through life, the perception of a deficit arose.

Deficit. It may not have been a medical, diagnosed 'deficit' but rather a word that came to reflect how she experienced herself in social situations. It became a lens through which she started to see her 'fit' in the world–especially in spaces where 'normal' or 'neurotypical' ways of being were most valued.

This difference became insidious, crouching in the corner of any experience that required social presence, logic, spatial awareness, stillness, or concentration. It fed itself on the energy of confusion until, one day, its precarious tower of questions became too visible, too loaded, too unstable to ignore.

Not knowing the right questions, the little girl kept trying to find answers everywhere. And although she achieved some things, how she went about them was so uncomfortable that any success paled into insignificance.

She believed herself to be blundering through life and that within her, there was something fundamentally 'wrong' or 'missing.' Because, if life was supposed to feel like treading water, surely, she should know about the depths beneath her?

Dear Reader, I invite you alongside me to view this childhood experience through a lens of self-compassion.

Had I, or someone around me, known the right questions to ask, perhaps I might have found the depths were not so deep after all and learned instead to swim. I'm beginning to feel compassion for the way undiagnosed ADHD has shaped my life, how it's felt like a lifelong act of 'making up for myself or overcompensating.

We are born whole human beings. Yet as

we step into the world, that wholeness can be called into question, especially when words like 'deficit' are used to describe parts of who we are. Thank goodness, there is a growing awareness that our systems and infrastructures must be adapted to reflect the diversity of everyone's experience in this world.

In light of those who work, advocate, and write on this subject, I feel hope. I am delighted to learn that awareness around the experience of living with ADHD and AuDHD is rising. So, hopefully, in the not-too-distant future, we may not need to dig so much for self-compassion. 'Dreamy little girls' and 'naughty little boys' will be celebrated for their 'varied attention'. The gifts of ADHD will be cultivated and, like tiny plants, offered the right conditions to thrive.

Presence

'Children have neither a past nor a future. Thus, they enjoy the present, which seldom happens to us.' – Jean de La Bruyère.

1971

I'm sitting on the grass in my childhood garden, around two years old, noticing its prickly touch on my legs. The sky resembles a school painting, flat, deep blue with a single, cloud-shaped cloud. I am surrounded by flowers–fat, pink, velvety mouths and rockets of red and purple. The tiny blue ones with yellow centres capture my heart – so many to love that I might fall in.

Joy is enormous in my tiny chest. Everything is... now! Puffs of warm air waft a heavy, clovey fragrance. A bumblebee, a fuzzy ball, hums as it works from flower to flower, and I wonder at the black dot moving on my toe and the tiny tickle it makes. My breath bursts forth, blending with the smells, colours, sounds, and sensations. I am immersed in the experience; it is part of me, and I of it.

Dear Reader, I invite you alongside me to view this childhood experience through a lens of self-compassion.

Vince Gowman writes, 'We can be present if only we allow ourselves to pause and appreciate the beauty and abundance of life once again, the same way we did when we were children.'

I can now begin to feel compassion for times, particularly during my teen years, when my soul's efforts to revisit the peace of my childhood garden brought me only to its gate, met with a jarring flashing sign of 'NO ACCESS'.

Much later, following an adulthood diagnosis of ADHD, I realised that when I give myself a break from trying so hard, the present moment 'arrives,' and the gate opens.

Perhaps, as adults with ADHD, we might all become curious about activities that deny us pause and recognise those that give us access to our present-moment awareness.

What's This?!

'It is a miracle that curiosity survives formal education.' – Albert Einstein.

1973

The living room has four 'things to do' corners. There are crayons and paper in one, books in another, beads and strings in the next, and play dough in the last. There is also a kitchen cupboard where I can pull all the plastic pots out, wash them up, and put them back in again. In the afternoon, we play a game of 'naming objects.' Mum lies on the sofa, and I wedge in at the end. I start with, 'What's this?' and Mum replies,

'That's a cushion.'

'That's a bookend.'

'That's a sweet wrapper.'

'That's a...'

Then we swap, and I become the namer of objects. The sophistication of this game grew over time to include spelling, using a thesaurus for word alternatives, and (still) my absolute favourite, rhyming.

There was tenderness in her recollections of my 'what's this?!' delivered with Jack Skellington-like wonder.

'You always wanted to learn, darling,' she would say.

Confident that I would surpass her academic expectations, my unfinished projects and oft-frequented C minus plateaus were befuddling to her.

Much later in life, on a day I brought my eldest son a blue iced drink and was on the brink of a parental-meltdown, I called my mum and wailed. She suggested I play the object game with him.

'It might slow him down and give you the break it gave me,' she said, her voice full of pride at having achieved the nearly impossible task of keeping me occupied.

Dear Reader, I invite you alongside me to view this experience through a lens of self-compassion.

Being a parent with undiagnosed ADHD and parenting a child with undiagnosed

ADHD was confusing. I often felt the urge to 'misbehave' alongside my children – I was once banned from being an attending parent on school trips for handing out imperial mints!

I can now find self-compassion for the ways my inability to be 'sensible' for long periods left me feeling inadequate and childlike among other parents and teachers. I studied to compensate. A degree is 'proof' of being a sensible person... isn't it? My 'Open Degree' is a broad hotchpotch of psychology modules with one common thread– trying to understand more about my way of being in the world.

Never did I try so hard as when my children were young, fuelled by a fear that I would be 'caught out' and they would be taken from my care. I feel compassion for that younger version of myself, who was good enough without trying so hard. And yet, it was only after exhausting every creative idea to keep my children occupied that I felt even vaguely accomplished. That it was 'my turn now' (to experience the relentless energy of 'a child-like you') seemed to hold karmic significance for my mum.

It seems appropriate that my counselling

specialism is self-compassion. Because, when I meet my younger self in the parents I now work with, I see how their new understanding of ADHD opens into empathy for their child's struggle and encourages them to find compassion around their own.

Otherwise... Something

'What a relief to discover that I wasn't really an idiot! I simply had a l earning disability.' – John H. Johnson.

1974

I'm at primary school and feel unchallenged by these first months of dressing up, name-writing, and painting. Unsure how to navigate friendship, I play 'mini teacher' with my peers.

Mummy still comes in to help me with my bows in the mornings, because they make me cry. When my teacher says to the class, 'Some people are so stupid and lazy they still get their mum to come in and tie their plimsole laces,' I know she means me.

Later in the year, I worry they will bring out the clock-face worksheets, the ones where we draw the hands-on. I copy Alison's work and feel bad, so give her pretty beads from my tin. But I always think I will be caught.

To my mum's delight, who had been part of the prevalent seventies trend of academic 'pushing' for pre-schoolers, it was decided that I would be advanced a year. Oddly, it was assumed that if kids were good at English, they were good at maths too!

But my screaming energy levels are met with a different attitude in this year group, and my reading level flattens to average. Sitting still and concentrating are prized, and 'moving around the classroom' is no longer tolerated.

In class, I keep giggling, then crying, just to get sent to the quiet room. And there is a 'timetable' thing that makes no sense. I watch my friends through the classroom divider window. Alison's blonde ponytail swings as she colours, and I feel out of place. Here, I am measured by small silver star stickers, and to get them, I must understand maths and how to tell the time, because 'otherwise...something.'

Dear Reader, I invite you alongside me to view this childhood experience through a lens of self-compassion.

I can now find compassion for my

younger self, who lived with the feeling that there was a danger inherent in not understanding things.

(Give me technology today, and up pops that same feeling!)

I believed that reaching a learning plateau meant I had to stop enjoying an activity, and that I must understand – given that the only reasons not to were stupidity or laziness.

While struggling, like gifts, belong to everyone, there are different kinds. The fact that nowadays children with ADHD might be helped to see both their unique struggles and blessings from early on makes hope swell in my heart!

The Axis that Connects

'Music is what feelings sound like.' – Georgia Cates.

1975

I'm sitting at a table in the living room of a house in Hatfield, England. Men with funny beards are playing music, and light from the bay window casts them into shadow. I'm colouring a picture and listening. The thumpy thumps inside the tune make me feel safe, and I'm able to comfortably stay still for a long time.

My dad was a friend, or maybe a roadie, for a psychedelic rock band Octopus. My memory holds him in giant headphones, singing Queen songs off-key at the top of his lungs, tears streaming down his face. ELO, Bread, and Yes were among the artists I was 'brought up on.'

We listened together, and I learned that music was what feelings sounded like for him. He wasn't a wordy man; songs were the axis that connected us.

Dear Reader, I invite you alongside me to view this childhood experience through a lens of self-compassion.

How precious, and painful, those songs would later become. Sadly, my father lost his life in an accident, and with practice, I can now begin to feel compassion for my younger self, who, within the pain of grief and whirls of confusion about my neurology, believed I would never again listen to our wonderful, shared tunes and rhythms without feeling the pain of loss. Their familiar patterns had helped me self-regulate, and without them, time gaped uncomfortably.

Kirsten Hutchinson writes, 'Music is rhythm, rhythm is structure, and structure is soothing to an ADHD brain struggling to regulate itself to stay on a linear path.'

So I turned to keeping busy as a way to self-regulate emotionally, starting projects I was capable of but could never seem to finish. That only deepened the confusion around my way of being! Now, in classrooms, children with ADHD are offered tools to emotionally regulate. Fidget toys are commonplace, and one earbud is not unheard of. What a changed world!

The Great Escape

'Every exit is an entry to
somewhere else' – Tom Stoppard.

1975

When I was changing for swimming yesterday evening, I whipped off my orange polo neck and pulled a muscle. Now, I must wear a neck brace. Made from rolled and flattened newspaper inside one of my mum's 'hint of tan' tights. It sounds crinkly, and my dad has folded it so that Concorde is taking off under my chin. Everybody laughs and now I can't do P.E. – I love climbing to the top of the ropes and think that even if they reached the sky, I wouldn't be scared.

Instead, I have to stay in the classroom and draw an object. Usually, I love drawing, but in this strange, still space. I can't choose an 'object,' so I start doodling instead. Suddenly, my page is full of patterns, and I worry. I can almost hear my teacher's voice, 'Why can't you just do what you were asked to do, Kathryn?'

A fizzy feeling starts in my head, and all I can think about is going home. Although the door has a high handle and a low one too, I could open it with my hand and foot by standing on a chair. The way home is easy.

When the police came, they called me a 'little escape artist.' And when my teacher said, 'What do you say, Kathryn?' I got to tell them 'My mum is an artist too!' But I couldn't get enough stars to stop my teacher from frowning, so I kept being extra helpful, hoping she'd think I was 'good' again.

I tear up while writing this anecdote because my grandson with ADHD has been excluded from class for being 'disruptive' and is quickly internalising that he is a 'bad boy.'

Following this incident, my confusion was immense. Despite my fawning (a lesser-known survival mechanism alongside fight, flight, and freeze), the teacher's continued frown told me that something about my whole way of being was unforgivable – that I could never 'make up for it'. Sometimes, I catch myself still trying.

Dear Reader, I invite you alongside me to view this childhood experience through a lens of self-compassion.

I now understand that my 'fizziness' was stress and hyperactivity. Being alone in an empty, silent, unstimulating classroom was daunting. I couldn't choose an object to draw (out of everything in the class!) because the task overwhelmed my executive function, and I couldn't even sit down properly, because I couldn't relax. Doodling repetitive patterns, something familiar, helped me emotionally regulate. But coming out of hyperfocus into that odd environment felt unsafe. I needed to get home.

Significant school changes punctuated my school years. Now, I feel self-compassion that the stress of being a 'new girl' put me in survival mode. Being hyper-aware (constantly scanning for danger) made it difficult to access my creativity (my safe place). Those were times I 'lost touch' with myself and became quickly overwhelmed.

I recently read that, from an evolutionary point of view, survival takes precedence over creativity. Stress hormones that prepare us for battle also interrupt the brain networks involved in creative thinking. Interestingly, offering simple, unchallenging creative activities to both adults and children can significantly reduce stress.

Winging it

'Success is stumbling from failure to failure with no loss of enthusiasm.' – Winston Churchill.

1976

My family has moved to a home in a Cambridgeshire village, where I joined its junior school at eight.

To my relief, I am 'put back.' My new classmates are the same age, and my difficulties with maths – among other things – go unnoticed. I feel free of something I don't have a word for, and it's wonderful. I'm also certain that this time, I'll understand maths if I try hard enough.

I take piano lessons with Mrs Bacon and do well until there are two rows of notes. Trying to remember the melodies doesn't quite work, because she always pulls a funny face at our next lesson and asks me why the tune has changed. Maths gets more complicated, so I start guessing the answers and making my numbers curly and pretty. The teacher asks what I'm doing, so I make my eyes big and stare until he turns round. Then, I put my school bag on my lap and cuddle it.

When Mum asks me to tell the time, the hands are never on the actual numbers, so I talk and talk with my eyes on the clock until they are. I worry about so many things, and I can't wait to go to the village secondary school. It will be somewhere I can start again. Again!

Dear Reader, I invite you alongside me to view this childhood experience through a lens of self-compassion.

The shame of not understanding was truly beginning to take hold, and I can now feel compassion for my younger self, who, believing that not understanding wasn't an option, began relying on smoke and mirrors as a way to cope.

As adults diagnosed with ADHD, our childhood confusion might slowly begin to realign as we form new understand-ings around our neurology. We might feel resistance at first – but perhaps, too, we might find some relief.

Willingly Captured

'Words make you think. Music makes you feel. A song makes you feel a thought.' – Yip Harburg.

1977

In the school hall, we're divided into two groups. Ours begins: 'Slow down; you move too fast; you got to make the morning last... just kicking down the cobblestones, looking for fun and feeling groovy.'

'Lalalalalalala... feelin' groovy,' comes the echo.

I love this song. I don't think much about the lyrics, but they go in. I need this song to last forever. Luckily, it's for a play, so we get to sing it over and over. And suddenly, I'm not the 'difficult' girl in the class anymore. Willingly captured within its patterns of notes and lyrics, I feel contained yet free to deviate slightly from its constraints.

The confusion comes later when I'm told

off in a maths lesson for still humming the tune, even though it was quietly, and seemed to make the class feel more 'possible.' Suddenly, I'm the most 'difficult' child again; as usual, I concentrate on making my numbers pretty, embellishing them with curls and flowers. My teacher tells me this is maths, not art, but I don't understand why it can't be both.

Dear Reader, I invite you alongside me to view this childhood experience through a lens of self-compassion.

For as long as I can remember, feeling able to wiggle safely along an otherwise straight line – to have 'growing room'– naturally activates my most capable self.

But when behaving 'appropriately' seems out of reach one day, and totally possible the next, it's a recipe for confusion at any age!

So often, I find compassion for my younger self in the confusion caused by my neurology. It feels momentous to realise that my intentions came from a place of 'trying to make sense of' and not 'trying to be disruptive.' This misunderstanding, that adults assumed I was trying to cause trouble, fed into my confusion about my intentions and eroded my self-esteem. But grown-ups knew everything, didn't they?

I feel compassion now that what instinctively supported my focus was deemed inappropriate. Perhaps listening to music while doing maths might have helped me emotionally regulate during those desperate, single-task moments.

My maths ability might not have improved had I been allowed to hum or listen to music in class. Yet, either one might have provided just enough stimulation to regulate my emotions, and helped me behave in line with my deepest intention: to be a 'good girl.'

Faces in the Wrong Places

'I memorise hair, jewelry, and favorite clothes. I recognise gaits, tics, and voices ... above all, I rely on context: a person of a certain type in our corridor is my colleague – but in the supermarket is probably a stranger.' – David Fine.

1977

It's a Saturday, and as usual, I'm in the local library with my mum, absorbed in a book called 'I am a Fox.' It's long and thin, and because it has to sit on the shelf sideways, it's always easy to spot. I have a favourite bean bag in the children's section, tucked in the corner beneath the portrait of a lady in a silver cardboard dress. The books I love most are on the shelves all around me. Mum says when I've selected a book, I should pop it under my bean bag. I know I'm allowed six, but I can only choose by doing eeny-meeny-miny-mo. Visiting this musty little flint building is the best morning of my week, and it's followed by a trip to the bun shop.

From far away, Mum is talking to me, and when I look up, she's standing with a lady in a pale pink coat and a fluffy hat.

'Look who's here,' I glance up. 'It's Mrs Miller, Katy!' Now Mum is nodding with her eyes alarmingly wide. Mrs Miller is my class teacher who has long brown hair, blue shoes with red laces, and a long beady necklace. I look again. It's hard to tell if it's her, and I search for clues. Then I spot her brown handbag, which goes next to her chair and is shiny like a conker. But I'm still not sure.

Dear Reader, I invite you alongside me to view this childhood experience through a lens of self-compassion.

I still need to see someone a dozen times before I feel confident it's them. While watching a film, I often interrupt with: 'Is that that woman or the other one' I rely on clues – usually clothing. But the only way to be certain is by comparison. Once, certain I saw someone who used to work with my dad, I chatted away until he said,

'You're very nice dear, but I don't know who you are.'

Maybe face blindness isn't a big deal, but as I write this, I realise it's definitely a 'thing.' As a teenager, my mum's friends often told her I had ignored them in town. But I hadn't recognised them – because I hadn't seen them! This fuelled my mum's perception of me as 'difficult.' I feel compassion now for the terrible awkwardness and confusion this accusation caused my younger self.

I've begun to be open about my face blindness, and it's surprising how many people say they don't 'do faces' either! And I continue to say 'hi' to anyone vaguely familiar, just in case!

Pushing Through

'A kite can't soar without some kind of force against it.' – Dakota Kirk.

1977, Onwards

I might be any age from eight onwards, and 'pushing through' is what life is about. I'm pushing through my confusion, cruel self-talk, and the emotions that arise when someone looks at me 'that way.' With gritted teeth, I'm pushing beyond my natural capabilities to prove myself worthy. There is another way to be. I know it, but it feels unthinkable. Because surely the 'other way' is what I have to fight. If I don't fight, I will have to give in. The question, though, is: give in to what?

Dear Reader, may I invite you alongside me to view this childhood experience through a lens of self-compassion.

Seeking self-worth from external sources can start early on for children with ADHD.

The approval of those around us matters at the survival level – no one wants to be thrown out of the 'pack.' But it matters, too, to teach our children how to understand and accept their own natural way of being. Doing so builds resilience in a world that still frowns on 'difference,' and helps us break the cycle of expecting neurodivergent people to mask who they are.

When a kite soars, the wind is the force against it. I acknowledge now that the forces I create to soar – to achieve anything 'proper'– can be unforgiving of my neurology. So I look to the nature of the wind to imagine what a kinder 'force against me' might feel like.

A kinder force would work with me, guide me upward gently, support me perfectly, and drop away from time to time so I might rest. Maybe an element of that kinder force is self-compassion.

Wherever I go, There I Am

'You believe that easily which you
hope for earnestly.' – Terence.

1978

I am around nine. Mum beckons me upstairs
to my room where she 'da das' with verve.
On my eiderdown are two synthetic pinafore
dresses, one burgundy, one green. Adorning
the fronts are oversized buttons, serving
no purpose. Hope transports me. These
dresses feel like instant allies; everyone is
wearing them. My new junior school in the
village has no uniform, and my own clothes
always seem wrong. But now, in these
dresses, I might finally belong – more like
everyone else, and somehow more OK.

Possibility surges through me. Future
school days feel suddenly smoothed of
confusion. I put off trying them on, but
my mum is insistent, and the spell breaks.
In the mirror, I look new. But inside, I'm
disappointed – because I still feel like me.

Dear Reader, I invite you alongside me to view this childhood experience through a lens of self-compassion.

My childhood self believed those dresses had the power to make her feel less different, and I can feel compassion for thinking I needed to be anything other than myself.

Might we hold to our hearts the impossible hopes of our younger selves in moments like this, and gently remind them they are enough?

Borders

'To read a book is to hold an entire world in the palm of your hand. That world is unique to you; no two readers can ever inhabit the same world.' – Arthur Schopenhauer.

1978

It's a particular kind of book – a possible one: heavy, hard-backed, and a little musty; its pages are rich with variety. Each picture, story, and poem are contained within a border. To slip between its pages is like pulling the bedcovers over my head during a terrible storm. Because somehow, these patterned boundaries offer me the safety of knowing exactly where to dive in.

I try not to recognise that I'm growing out of this book's stories. I begin making my own version in scrapbooks, glueing in more age-appropriate, copied-out stories, poems, and passages from other books, all using the same bordered format. I fill the gaps with my own poetry and pictures. I get a 'poem head' at night that won't stop rhyming.

I'm in love with stories. I always need to read the first page of a long book many times, because it feels too exciting to start, and I seem to read without reading. Then suddenly, I'm in. From morning to night, into the night, at the dinner table, even reading in the bath, the book wrapped in a clear plastic bag – the book that is, not me! Mum and Dad call me a bookworm, which means something good. But if I'm told to stop and do something else, especially have dinner or go out, it's awful. Uncomfortable and cold. Like how I imagine being born might feel, and my shoulders hunch up just thinking about it.

Dear Reader, I invite you alongside me to view this childhood experience through a lens of self-compassion.

I feel such gratitude that I was read to from babyhood and later held in safety, terrified, while the wolf gobbled Red Riding Hood's grandmother and Bluebeard's wife attempted to scrub blood from a key. Later, I read 'Storytelling with Children' by Nancy Mellon. Truth blends with magic in her work, reacquainting me with why I love stories so deeply.

Mellon writes, 'children look for the love

and respect you have for yourself, and your experiences.'

So maybe beginning to reframe the stories of my childhood (which I now share with my children and grandchildren) nurtures all of us. Through these anecdotes, triumph and disaster can be – in the words of Kipling – treated 'just the same' for they are indeed imposters in a world that serves these extremes as polarities in either or soup. Within all experiences, there may be value: courage and hope, wisdom and fear.

A particular favourite is the one about my fourteen-year-old self, having lost her purse along with her return ticket, trying to get a free bus ride home by saying I was thirteen. I was asked for my birth date and was unable to do the sum; I gave the year, which made me fifteen! Oh! The fear of being stranded, and the courage it took to lie. Oh! The hope of being believed. And oh! The lessons around honesty, and the learning to never tell an untruth beyond my ability to do the maths! It's a heady blend of feelings, and the grandkids always come closer at the part where I'm squirming... Will I be 'found out?' Worse, I am found out. But I am also understood and pitied.

Told simply to 'just get on.' Triumphant disaster and disastrous triumph, perhaps?

Trying on a Way

'Curiosity is one of the great secrets of happiness.'
– Bryant H. McGill.

1978

My cousins are visiting from Australia, and I feel magic in the air. Ali wears a cornflower blue dress on lightly tanned skin. Her accent is otherworldly and, when spoken into the still air of our small English village home, it's thrilling! I need to see what happens if I talk this way. 'Being Australian' gives me a new feeling, and something about it feels safer. There's a knack for speaking this way. I practice noticing how 'a' sounds different- more like 'e.'

Perhaps shifting my focus from what I said to how I said it moved my fear away from the part of me that sensed I often said the 'wrong thing.' It becomes a homespun Aussie twang that carries on long after my cousin's visit until it morphs into (thinking back and cringing) something

Dame Edna Everage-esque... and starts making people laugh.

Dear Reader, I invite you alongside me to view this childhood experience through a lens of self-compassion.

Now, conscious of an implicit childhood belief that there must be another, more acceptable way to be me, I can begin to feel self-compassion around this experience. Low self-esteem and ADHD can go hand in hand when we get lost in self-doubt. While writing this right now, I can feel self-doubt creeping in.

Will this book resonate with anyone?...

Is it rubbish?... Probably.

Will I be laughed at? Arrested?

I am aware that I rely on my hyperfocus and wonder if it is somehow cheating if I don't write from my 'thinking' mind. Do I even have one?! Working this way is exciting, but the hyperactive buzzing that allows me to sense what connects, and to see from different angles, is exhausting.

Perhaps we begin to heal our low self-esteem as we begin to understand our neurology and cultivate self-compassion around the things we can't change. Maybe, in time, we might even come to see value in them.

Found in Words

'Creativity is just connecting things. When you ask creative people how they did something, they feel a little guilty because they didn't really do it. They just saw something. It seemed obvious to them after a while.' – Steve Jobs.

1979

At ten, I learned how never to finish a book. In the last chapter of the current book, I would read the first chapter of the next, thus avoiding the feeling of a massive hole opening beneath me. A book is a whole world; I don't want to be anywhere else. So I made sure there was always somewhere safe to go.

I love to write poems; they are the only thing I can finish. They feel complete, like a song or a picture. I feel like I'll explode with excitement when words fall in tune with each other. But my friend is cross, because she never gets a poem on the wall, and I always do. But it was easy, and I begin to wonder whether I've somehow cheated.

The feeling I get with maths, though, never changes. It's sticky and scary and feels like being frowned upon does. Dad tries to teach me maths at home. He shouts at me, telling me something must be wrong with my brain if I can't understand this simple sum. He says it's easy; I could be a nurse, and he would be proud of me then.

But when we visit the hospital for mum's joints, I see charts with numbers and pots with measurements on the side, and I'm not so sure. Still, the nurses wear uniforms, so maybe if I wore a uniform and I blended in, my brain might work properly. Maybe then I'd be OK with shoelaces, and with the kind of watch you have to read upside down.

Dear Reader, I invite you alongside me to view this childhood experience through a lens of self-compassion.

When I showed even the sniff of ability for something, my mum would say, 'Oooo, maybe you can be a ....' This litany of future possibilities became pressure over time, culminating in many 'we would be proud of you if...' statements: if you were a nurse, a teacher, a solicitor - a 'profes-sional.' My poetry was never mentioned in a career context and felt more like a party trick. I always sensed that my parents' enthusiasm around what I would do eclipsed their enthusiasm for who I already was, as a being. It felt as though I had already failed at personhood, and that unless I understood maths, they would never be proud of me.

I feel compassion towards my younger self, where I longed for my heart and soul to be accepted, but thought I would have to fulfil an expectation first. Taking my parents' conditions of worth as my truth became clear when I began studying to be a counsellor, a 'professional.' Exploring this career choice during my training was quite revealing.

Perhaps my parents were 'looking forward,' beyond their parenting of this 'difficult child' to a time when having a professional job meant she would be a professional person too – aka not such a 'difficult' one. I smile a little, writing this, remembering my mum saying, 'You do realise that you'll have to start doing things properly when you become a nurse/ teacher/solicitor.'

Maybe they hoped my chosen profession would finally 'contain me?' I'm glad to have teased out my truth from this mess – or is it my mess from their truth? Human 'beingness' eclipses human 'doingness.' The two are not mutually exclusive, but they frequently merge a treat during creative activity!

Masking is Multi-Tasking

'Aspects of masking have become second nature, and the effort to unmask can be on par with what masking once felt like!' – Katy.

When I put my head on the table in history class, the teacher taps my shoulder. I don't tell her I can understand better with my eyes closed, because she'll give me a funny look. Adults often give me that same look, and I'm beginning to know what face I need to wear so they don't. But it feels still and uncomfortable. So when I get home, I take it off and my mum gets cross. She says, 'I bet you don't talk like that to other people!' And she's right.

Dear Reader, I invite you alongside me to view this childhood experience through a lens of self-compassion.

I still sometimes mask 'whole body calm,' but it feels like spacewalking. I feel compassion for everyone with ADHD who masks just to be 'less annoying.' Also, it's often only when a child gets home that they feel safe to unmask.

For years, I thought learning to be other than you are, along with always being uncomfortable was something everyone had to do. But slowing my speech and not fidgeting, at the same time as curbing impulsivity and restlessness as well as hiding emotional volatility, was a lot to pull off in one go. And, unsurprisingly, something always 'slipped through.' Every day I felt back to square one.

I thought it was, without question, beneficial to other people if I wasn't 'myself'. But I've come to realise this belief only reinforces the expectation that neurodivergent people will squeeze themselves into a neurotypical shape, normalizing an intolerance of difference. Self-acceptance begets acceptance. And often, it begins with us.

I'd love to say that being diagnosed with ADHD in adulthood allowed me to unmask. But in truth, some aspects of masking have become second nature, and the effort to unmask can feel just as intense as the effort it once took to mask!

Doesn't Everyone?

'My day starts backward. I wake up tired
and go to bed wide awake.' Anon.

1979

I'm going back to school later this evening for a gymnastics event. Mum gives me a sandwich. But after sandwiches, the top of my stomach hurts and looks like a funny square shape under my leotard. I start getting a bit scared to eat.

When my mind gets busy at night, I get up and do cartwheels and backbends, handstands, and balances in the living room. Doesn't everyone? Then I return to bed and read until I fall asleep.

Dear Reader, I invite you alongside me to view this childhood experience through a lens of self-compassion.

Much later, bread is replaced with something gluten-free, and gymnastics with yoga poses. I still practice while the kettle boils, and sometimes, when my legs get restless at night, I have a little boogie in the living room.   Doesn't everyone?

Even now, I sometimes go to bed hungry because I can't always distinguish between feelings of hunger, anxiety and excitement. When I tell my son (who also has ADHD) that I need to 'go running or something,' he tells me:

'You can't outrun your ADHD brain.'

And I tell him, 'I can try.'

As a child, eating grounded me, but I didn't want to feel grounded during the day. A gluten intolerance made my body feel dull, highlighting my busy mind, which I liked to constantly match with movement. I feel compassion for my younger self, who went on to believe food was 'the enemy.'

Eating 'healthily' can be challenging for people with ADHD. Despite our good intentions, food so often involves decision-making, and our executive functions can feel defeated before we've even started eating. It might even be self-compassionate when we reach for something 'easy,' but our self-berating can be too strong to allow us to see that.

AuDHD makes both the decision-making and the sensory aspects of eating feel like a jarring task switch—something I put off again and again. Porridge, eggs, or bananas, with their gentle flavours and satisfying simplicity, have become my go-to options.

So, wherever our neurodivergence has brought us in our relationship with food, recognising our patterns and embracing them, on some level, can be a deeply self-compassionate step.

Worth the Gamble

'People who have low self-esteem might not even know they have low self-esteem.' – Yong Kang Chan.

1979

Around nine, I am learning that what I say cannot then be unsaid. I ask question after question and spill secrets the moment they are told. On some level, I have clocked that this changes the way people see me, but if something feels not OK, I can't gauge how not OK it is. And to be the only bearer is unbearable.

Long after my peers had grasped it, I was still unable to weigh this particular kind of importance. I began to notice that my outspokenness earned a few laughs. So, I slipped into friendship groups through the back door of humour. And although it sometimes got me into trouble, the hope of being included for being funny and quirkily honest – always more likely than being properly understood – usually felt worth the gamble.

Even into my forties, I was still considered a bit of a 'loose cannon' (Ow!) until my understanding of appropriateness and consequence fully developed. Bantering back with a joke had become my conversational style because being taken seriously for being 'funny' was better than what happened when I was serious. But eventually, my faith in my emotional memory (my gut feelings) became strong enough to trust.

Dear Reader, I invite you alongside me to view this childhood experience through a lens of self-compassion.

I recognise that self-regulation took me longer than my peers. Hyperactivity, coupled with the ways ADHD impacted my executive functions, I found it hard to gauge situations requiring decision-making, including what to say and when. This gave rise to comments about being 'childish,' and I now feel compassion for the younger me, who used humour as the safest form of expression and believed she always had to 'perform.' Maybe it's interesting that one of the places I feel safest is on stage, singing. Looking at people chatting at their tables, I often think – 'that looks like really hard work!'

Capping off something serious with humour to make light of pain is still my tendency. But lately, being 'the quiet one' in a gathering saves me from what I now recognise to be social exhaustion – we have a 'social battery!' Who knew? I can feel compassion for the times I approached social situations full of joy and verve, only to leave disorientated and tearful.

I'm glad, however, to see the funny side of the human condition. And nowadays, it feels safer to be serious too – a balance, perhaps?

But when I notice someone with ADHD neurology being 'the clown,' it resonates deeply. Reminds me of the immense weight of the traits I was trying to hide, just to feel acceptable.

Going Off Piste

'Perhaps some things are not as 'off course'
as 'of course'!' – Anon.

1979

Aged ten, I have been given a small tapestry kit. A bright orange deer is printed on the woven fabric. Thrilled with anticipation, I begin going over and over with the orange wool – over and over and over. There are instructions, but as usual, I 'do my own thing,' and soon there's no way back. When I start going wrong at the front, I try to make up for it on the back, pulling the wool straight across to fill missed stitches and hoping for the best. I begin to 'double up' the body for a more 3D appearance, and for hours, the world shrinks to the size of my needlepoint.

When I run out of orange wool, the world zooms back out to full size. Suddenly, the tapestry looks nothing like the picture on the box. I feel dread... panic! My mum can't understand why I would 'ruin it on purpose, like everything else,' and I half believe I have. The mound of orange lurks atop white linen in my mother's sewing chest for years, a fish finger on ice representing every unfinished thing I ever started.

Dear Reader, I invite you alongside me to view this childhood experience through a lens of self-compassion.

In the nineteen seventies, ADHD neurology in girls wasn't on many people's radar. In this scenario where I'm having difficulty following instructions, my under-stimulated ADHD brain needed to make the craft more exciting, so I 'did my own thing,' becoming happily hyper-focused and losing sight of the bigger picture (albeit one of a deer).

The idea that I might 'ruin it on purpose' was painful and confusing, and now my heart feels heavy for my younger self. Knowing I was capable, my mum drew an understandable conclusion, given that this was not my first project that had gone 'off-piste.'

Decades later, it's still the same – of course! Isn't tweaking a sewing pattern or recipe what makes it exciting!? And lately, I'm finding that giving myself leeway is what makes beginning things possible. While there is no guarantee of the outcome – and there is often disappointment – it is the 'way of doing' that brings me joy.

Perhaps I can begin to offer myself compassion when my undone things make me disapprove of myself and disrupt my inner harmony.

Remember This, Remember This

'Life gives you plenty of time to do whatever you want to do if you stay in the present moment.' – Deepak Chopra.

1979

I'm ten. I still can't tell the time on a clock, but I can stretch it by saying to myself, 'Remember this, remember this.' If I keep saying it and notice every detail, I get to 'stay,' and a 'perfect moment' can go on and on. If I forget to do this, time seems to pass in chunks. Sometimes, while reading a book, it suddenly gets dark outside, and I always miss my turn when playing games.

I try to shrink time in maths by saying 'faster, faster,' but this never works. Instead, it goes so slowly that I have to put my head in my arms on the desk and go to sleep. I know my times tables up to twelve because Mum helps me say them in a sort of song-poem, and each has its own rhythm. I don't really know what they mean, though.

Twisty questions like 'A man goes into a shop and buys a bun for 50p, it costs 27p, so how much change does he have?' make me dizzy. If I'm asked to repeat the question, I just keep really, really still and hardly breathe until my eyes get big and fill, and they turn away. But it's not a problem with my memory. I can remember things from ages ago – whole songs from adverts and being in my pushchair wearing a pale blue raincoat that smelled like a beachball.

Dear Reader, may I invite you alongside me to view this childhood experience through a lens of compassion.

Understanding the link between time, presence, and memory recently brought a big 'ah hah' moment. So that's why I lose things all day long! As a child, I struggled to stay present and felt confused that my way of being seemed to make time (and objects) disappear.

Although hyperfocus and zoning out were traits beyond my understanding, their consequences in everyday environments made me feel shame. I can feel compassion for the fear and belief held by my younger self that one day I wouldn't 'be there' when it mattered, and something awful might happen.

This feeling of dread weaves its own thread through my memories of childhood. But with new understandings around my neurology, I can engage with memories 'apart' from those happenings and discover different, sensory threads of sounds, tastes and smells.

It's helped to examine the background of childhood photographs, prompting me to recognise the people, things and places that I loved, and gently reawaken forgotten threads. Perhaps most wonderful of all are the patterns and colours of nineteen-seventies wallpaper!

jhjh and fgfg

'When your room is clean and uncluttered, you have no choice but to examine your inner state.' – Marie Kondo.

1979

I'm ten. My godmother, Claire, has moved to our village. I frequently pedal to her cottage on my bicycle, and she teaches me to knit. I am right-handed; she is left. She tells me to do what she is doing but around the other way. I'm confused by her adamance that this is easy, and thrown by her shortening patience. My head fizzes. I cry. Claire doesn't know me like this. I used to be just a 'visitor' in her life, and now I can't escape being known. Something is spoiled.

Claire unearths her typewriter. It is beautiful. It lives in a pristine case, and I devote a whole summer holiday to sitting in Claire's minimalist living room, learning to touch type. I am contained, loving that Pitman's book stands up on its own and prescribes that I 'jhjh' and 'fgfg.'

I love and hate how Claire's tidiness creates an 'other dimension' that feels impossible at home – something spacious and surprisingly peaceful inside me.

Just last week, I had watched my mum scrabbling frantically in her handbag for a lost key and felt repulsed by the scene, then guilt-wracked at mentally comparing her to Claire. Mum is super-creative. Everything in our home feels softened with her love, from the painted daisies on our navy-blue kitchen cupboards, to the tiny painted mouse running along to its painted mousehole on the skirting.

Words like quirky and fascinating, dreamy, and sensitive, which were surely compliments, were incongruous with the deep frown embedded in Claire's tone, one that lingered over her description of my mother's way of being in general.

Later, it was my turn to be frowned upon. And in time, of course, I became my mother in so many ways, delighting my children with jungle bedroom walls, flour bombs and the glitter bits from Christmas we were still discovering in June. A version of shabby chic already existed in my head before its commercial debut in 1989 and made allowances for the decadence of just about anything. I was delighted when a sofa with a questionable arm eventually became the chaise lounge it was destined to be!

Dear Reader, may I invite you alongside me to view this childhood experience through a lens of compassion.

I feel compassion that my young adult self would become as uncomfortable in her own home as Mum had seemed when Claire visited. But Claire's snipes about mother-daughter similarities helped to reveal to me, at last, my tired projections onto Mum about the disorderliness I felt self-destined for.

There really was something about Claire's minimalist space that created spaciousness within me. My childhood home was too visually stimulating for this to 'happen.' But realizing I can't reorganise my mind's natural way by organizing a drawer, I now find my spaciousness by looking at naturally minimalistic things, like the sky, or visiting a coffee shop for half an hour.

Incidentally, I did try the Marie Kondo

'perfectly rolled' clothes drawer. Proud to report to my daughter I had kept it 'just so' for months, she looked inside and proclaimed, 'But these are the things you never wear!'

I didn't want to 'turn out like my mother' (what a child does), but I have. And apart from the crappy joints, I wouldn't change it for the world!

Something Tilts a Bit

'A friend is someone who understands your past, believes in your future, and accepts you today the way you are.' – Anon.

1979

I've been writing a song. Putting music to words tickles my brain into a strange stillness, and I've only just realised that lyrics are the same as poetry!

Alarmed because what felt like fifteen minutes was actually three hours, my heart jolts. I know I have forgotten something. The fact that it's Saturday flutters at the edge of my awareness. But it can't be, can it? Dazed, something tilts a bit, and dread panic begins in my chest.

Only yesterday, we had been anticipating the best time. Debbie told me her mum has made a lucky dip, and that one of the gifts was a wooden whistle. So if I felt something long and thin, I should choose it – but pretend to be surprised. In my ten-year-old way, I conclude that I am a rubbish friend and a horrid person, and I try to determine whether forgetting is the same as when time just… slips away. I was deeply sad, but not just about missing the party.

Dear Reader, may I invite you alongside me to view this childhood experience through a lens of compassion.

The way that letting someone down reached into my throat and squeezed my heart is unforgettable. But no longer is it unforgivable. I now have a wrist alarm and calendar for brain backup, and accept that I need them. Children don't know about calendars; children with ADHD inevitably lose mornings to hyperfocus.

That Saturday afternoon, my shame rounded me from all sides. It felt thick, like guilt, and I stood in Debbie's shoes and 'went through' her disappointment repeatedly. Similar haunting happenings contributed to my blossoming reputation for unreliability, and self-berating became my everyday self-speak. I had already internalised the idea that allowing time to 'slip' was 'thoughtless' (unless I had something to show for it). As a result, I'm still frequently an over-doer, and as much as I love engaging with you, Dear Reader, writing this book exemplifies overdoing, following an already busy day.

Only recently can I feel compassion for the decades it took to become a 'true friend' to myself, one who understands my past, believes in my future and accepts who I am today.

More and more, though, taking time out from doing to simply being, matters. Sometimes, when I stop, there's the realisation that the 'there' I've been trying to get to all day is actually 'here and now', in my dog's smile, and the comfort of my home.

A No Particular Summer Night's Dream

'In each of us is another whom we do not know. He speaks to us in dreams and tells us how differently he sees us from the way we see ourselves.' – Carl Jung.

1980

Before my adulthood diagnosis, dreams were a frantic scrabbling that mirrored, twisted, and magnified my daytime experiences tenfold. Typically nightmarish, they seemed to solidify my negative feelings about myself. A recurring theme was that I had buried someone. Running through this was a dread feeling and confusion about what I had 'done,' and that it was only a matter of time before I was 'caught.' In another, my efforts – in vain – to make an appointment on time, and a scenario where I am trying to explain myself to a disgruntled colleague, run concurrently. I feel confident and articulate, but something is off. Familiarly, belief in me collapses, first in the listener's eye, then in my chest. I sense a meaning, but it's vague and smoky.

Dear Reader, may I invite you alongside me to view this experience through a lens of self-compassion.

I was so far from feeling I was allowed to be 'myself' in the world that I might have found its softness suspicious, had self-compassion met me in those childhood dreams.

The burial dream stopped the moment I embraced having ADHD. Maybe having this explanation for the aspects of self that I'd needed to 'bury' meant that I felt safe enough to be unearthed?

As adults diagnosed with ADHD, when daytime confusions and anxieties follow us into our dreams, and anxious dreams follow us into our days, perhaps self-compassion means more purposefully finding havens of rest during our waking hours.

Faux Pas

'People can be at their most vulnerable but still tenacious at the same time.' – Toni Bernhard.

1980

I go with my mum to an office called 'the solicitor.' It's all very formal. The man looks busy and sensible in the way my parents like. And there are so many books! Mum is dressed like a liquorice allsort in pink and black. I stand by her chair and (so he doesn't think I am like I am) earnestly tell the man behind the massive desk that I would like to do soliciting when I get older. When he smiles at me kindly, I guess it must be in praise of my career choice.

Dear Reader, may I invite you alongside me to view this childhood experience through a lens of self-compassion.

This faux pas later mortified my younger self, and it took years for me to appreciate the humour, because the joke was entirely on me. Children with ADHD can often feel 'left behind' in their understanding. Their efforts to 'keep up' tend to reveal things about which they are naïve, leading to sudden bouts of shame and overwhelm. In trying to show maturity, I had revealed my naivety – something that only recently sits comfortably with me as 'all part of the journey.' I have to concede that most world news and the lives of celebrities are still completely off my radar.

Regarding careers, I take my work as a counsellor for neurodivergent adults seriously, but I've never held down a 'company' job in a 'traditional' (neurotypical) way.

Over time, I've noticed it's not uncommon for neurodivergent people to move sideways rather than straight up in their careers, nurturing their inexhaustible search for interest and building a diverse range of skills.

So, let's throw the lens of compassion wide open, to include every neurodivergent person who has found the world of work a struggle to negotiate, particularly those who find 'holding down a job' challenging, or find themselves working in ways that make them physically, spiritually, emotionally or financially vulnerable.

Forging ahead in creative, untraditional ways while simultaneously using unkind words to describe ourselves seems to be a 'thing' for some people with ADHD. But if a self-deprecating mantra plays on a loop and becomes our motivation, we may not be able to appreciate our small, meaningful achievements.

A string of lights will shine in the formation where we place them. Practising the use of kinder, softer words in place of harsh self-talk can light new patterns – new neural pathways to self-compassion that offer softer feelings around our humanness.

I will never forget the day my brain said 'no' to self-berating and offered me a kind thought instead. The redirection felt physical.

Safe from Chaos

'Ideas excite me, and as soon as I get excited, the adrenaline gets going, and the next thing I know, I'm borrowing energy from the ideas themselves.'
– Ray Bradbury.

1980

I'm eleven. I've missed my usual toast for breakfast, but it's nice not to have the horrid stomach that makes me breathless, and then need to undo the button on my skirt. Before long, I feel whizzy, the world falls away, and I begin writing poems that seem to link into each other.

I'm using hunger's adrenaline release to fuel my creativity and get into hyperfocus. This soothes my chaotic mind, but I'm getting into deep water.

Now scared to eat unless it's just before bedtime, a teacher speaks to my mum about me being 'anorexic.' Suddenly, the way I had found to make the pain go away, and creativity possible, was something horrible I was 'doing to myself.'

Because there was no language around this kind of thing, the intrusion of adults was clumsy. My desperate mum didn't know where to start and usually began baking. But telling her that her cakes hurt my tummy was super tricky. Unfortunately, I got pretty unwell before discovering I was gluten intolerant, and the memory of the pain of 'bloating' still makes me feel a little panicky about feeling 'full.'

Dear Reader, may I invite you alongside me to view this childhood experience through a lens of compassion.

Several nasty things happened to my body when I restricted my eating. I won't share them, as you can probably imagine. But I can find self-compassion in having experienced the feeling of being blamed for something I knew I couldn't help. Even now, I work better on an empty stomach, though I stay mindful of hunger pangs.

Pervasive feelings of shame and confusion around eating can be part of a childhood with undiagnosed AuDHD – it could easily be a book of its own! My female clients in particular present this duo over and over. And when they are ready to visit their childhood selves through the lens of self-compassion, their emotional healing can positively impact their current relationship with food and eating.

Many people with AuDHD 'graze,' finding that responding to hunger works better than to the clock. It's common to hear a client say they eat once a day because the sensory experience of food is too disturbing.

It took a long time to realise I had sensory issues around food. It might be termed 'disordered eating,' given that breakfast, lunch, and dinner are considered 'normal.' Although reaching for the first available – not always healthy – snack is likely, perhaps this might just as correctly be called 'eating in tune with our neurology'?

Wishy-Washy

'It may be difficult for her to make firm decisions on even simple tasks so that she seems wishy-washy and indecisive.' – TotallyADD.

1980

Turning eleven comes with a growing awareness of being disapproved of. This 'comes on' suddenly. It emanates from friends' parents who greet me at their front doors, dull toned with a 'not you again' expression that blends all their faces into one. I know I pressed the doorbell for a long time, but that's because I can't hear it from outside.

The word 'disruptive' works itself into the mix, and making eye contact, especially with adults, becomes excruciating. Just anticipating the requirement to do so makes my eyes stream embarrassingly. I feel there's something different about me, and it is closing my joy and confidence down. Dark shadows are appearing in corners where understanding needs to be.

One friend tells me her dad said I'm not trustworthy because I can't look him in the eye. Another says her mum thinks my mum is 'wishy-washy'. It's the first time I've heard an expressed opinion about one of my parents. This woman is a teacher. I know this makes her a plausible person; my mum can see I know this. My whirling, loving, artistic mother is despairing as the timing of our roast dinner in a pre-micro-wave world defeats her. Scratching like a DJ at the hob, she says, 'The woman is hard. She puts her career first and wears the trousers.'

But this doesn't make sense. Mum has always worn trousers and had a career before having me, and I just need to know what 'wishy-washy' means!

Dear Reader, I invite you alongside me to view this childhood experience through a lens of self-compassion.

That particularly unkind description of a neurodivergent person really upsets me, on my mum's behalf. Perhaps it digs into the edginess and vulnerability of my 'not quite getting it.'

'It,' here meaning the 'doing of life.'

Around this age, a bright strand within my tapestry's thread stands out in contrast, and I begin living at awkward angles to conceal it.

I can feel a tenderness towards my younger self, who, while unwittingly just being a girl with ADHD neurology, is hyper-aware that the meaning of 'wishy-washy' might hold the answer to something she doesn't yet know the question for.

As adults with ADHD, knowing that it tends to run in families may support our process of finding clues to our heredity that support our feelings of self-worth. I didn't have to look far, and now I can laugh a little. Will those dials ever correspond to the hob plates? Never!

Congruence

'Your private self must become the same as your public self.' – John Kuypers.

1981

I'm twelve. Mum sits me down and tells me I must be friendly towards our neighbour, Vicky. I plead that I can't pretend. Something so strong courses through me. A knowing that I can't explain.

I have to write a poem immediately. It's about a butterfly being eaten by a fox. Mum frowned and told me I didn't write it. Then, in the next breath, she tells me what a nuisance it is that she has to keep doing things for Vicky.

Vicky makes me cringe, and I scowl hard when she leans into me and says, 'We like to keep Mum busy, don't we.' It's not a question, but the answer comes anyway. Somehow, I already ran Mum off her feet – without even trying.

Dear Reader, may I invite you alongside me to view this childhood experience through a lens of compassion.

Having to pretend we like someone we don't feels inauthentic. Children suffer confusion when asked to be inauthentic. Learning the skill of being tact develops around the age of six to eight, but I'm sure it came later for me. For a while, disliking someone without expressing it was impossible, long past the age when that was socially acceptable.

When studying to be a therapist, I realised just how confused I'd been. I'd never learned that it was OK to privately discern between who I did like and who I didn't, or that I could be honest with myself. Offering everyone unconditional positive regard, I had absorbed my mum's people-pleasing tendencies and was naïve to the idea that people could have hidden agendas. It was liberating to begin trusting my gut feelings and knowing that my relationship choices could become healthier by regularly 'checking in' with myself.

I still get caught out sometimes. But now, I recognise that anyone I feel the need to 'fawn to' is probably someone I should spend less time with. This oft-mis-understood fight-or-flight response is natural. Our social survival depends on inclusion, but our personal wellbeing is just as important. So it matters to keep 'checking in' with ourselves.

It's Not About Socks

'To be yourself in a world that is constantly trying to make you something else is the greatest accomplishment.' – Ralph Waldo Emerson.

1981

Being someone else looks easier, but I can't quite fathom why. For a while now, my almost-teenage self has been convinced that wearing bright white socks is the difference.

I read a story about a girl who wishes she was someone else. There follows a magical changing of minds and bodies. But being inside this other girl feels strange because she doesn't appreciate the same things.

I don't want to be someone else, and I genuinely love how I experience life's bounty. It's too exciting sometimes. I am the musical nun with her favourite things! Books and nature, the smell of other people's houses, colours and skies, gymnastics and jumble sales, music and yes, actually, warm woollen mittens (so long as they aren't itchy) are a few of mine.

But at school, the white-socked girls tug at my ease of being. Significantly stiller and quieter, they can work through all of their classes without planning various escapes to the loo or beneath the desk to rescue a rubber. Their pencil cases have everything they need, and their writing is always the same. I keep having to borrow pens, and because all my exercise books get progressively messier, I try filling them quickly to start anew. These girls don't have to keep starting anew – I know it! Nor do they keep asking the teacher to 'say that again, please' or spend half a lesson talking, leg-swinging, balancing back on two chair legs (my favourite) or doodling, and the other half with their head on the table.

My maths difficulties are eventually discovered, and my dad says this was 'my last chance.' I had started out with so many hopes. During the summer holidays, I had learned many French words, lured by this new, shiny language and curious about the French grandmother I'd never met. But it's the middle of the second year now, and I've fallen behind. I was fine until we moved on to verbs. Something familiar sits thickly in my throat.

In English and Art, time goes so fast that coming out of the classroom gives me the odd 'coming back into the world' feeling I get after reading a whole book or exiting the cinema. But in maths, it's as though I can see the teacher's lips moving, and nothing means anything. It happens in French now, too.

The school has a new music block. I spend all my lunchtimes writing songs. I can't face lunch and feel all whizzy. Mum boils my socks, so they are bright white. But it makes no difference at all.

Dear Reader, may I invite you alongside me to view this childhood experience through a lens of compassion.

This 'other way of being' fascinated me, and I knew those girls were getting it right on a level I couldn't. Not just the learning part, but something else. Later, 'Get it right' became the self-berating mantra of my early teens.

I had formed an idea of the 'right way to be,' and my authentic self didn't measure up. I feel compassion for my younger self, thinking it looked easier to be someone else. Of course, it did! I only saw them. I didn't experience being them.

An ADHD diagnosis, and accepting I likely had ASD traits too, was the catalyst that enabled me to move into a place of genuine self-understanding. It allowed me to embrace my humanness as an OK thing and begin a journey towards self-compassion.

Regarding difficulties with maths, it only ever occurred to me to hide it. I feel compassion for my younger self, who, terrified of being 'found out,' welcomed every school change like a safe hiding place.

It's not unusual for girls with ADHD to reject authenticity in favour of more socially acceptable ways of being. After all, everyone needs to survive in their social environment. Maybe, as we begin to embrace our ADHD way of being, a glimmer of the blissful authenticity of young childhood might begin to feel accessible again.

Part Two:

The Huge Wordless Question

We Had Been the Same Once

'She may experience a wide range of emotions that go along with the biological, cognitive, and social changes that are taking place.' – Keath Low.

1983

One Sunday, my dad – a fireman impatient for a call out – threw up his hands during a roast chicken dinner and said,

'Listen, family. There just aren't enough fires in a village!'

That summer holiday of my fifteenth year, we moved once again from the sleepy village to the market town of my early childhood.

Suddenly, I am someone else, somewhere else. If my body is going to change like this, I need to be at home, in the village where I am written into its cottage walls and windows.

Feeling both confined and exposed, my behaviour is volatile; my parents tell me not to 'create.' I'm only vaguely aware of forming dangerous friendships and falling behind at school during a crucial time. I never seem to feel 'easy' inside and trying takes everything I've got.

Dear Reader, may I invite you alongside me to view this childhood experience through a lens of compassion.

Among oddly different versions of my first school playmates, familiar names belong to unfamiliar faces. The children who once filled my dreams and had settled into being memories were suddenly revived. My compassion arises remembering the feeling I had when I opened my cupboard and saw my childhood things. How I turned Buttons, my rag doll, towards the wall so she couldn't see me. We had been the same once.

In my parents' words was the truth of what I needed to do: create. Filled with fear and now in survival mode, my awareness was too heightened for creativity, and everything I loved doing was suddenly beyond my reach.

They Sort of Shine

'There's a resonance inside us, a sense of who we are. We're a multi-bodied traveller. We're an essence. We're a feeling, an awareness that has an ancient existence.' – Frederick Lenz.

1980

I think Claire has a personality because she is the same way with everyone. What she'd do in any given situation is obvious. I'm confused as to why I don't seem to have that sort of 'definiteness.' It's not just a Claire thing, either. Some children in the class are similar. Sometimes, pretending I'm Claire when making a decision makes it easier.

I hate when people say things I do are 'youish' because that's not my personality. 'Youishness' is what I want to stop, so I might discover my true personality!

Youish things just happen. Like the massive excitement about colour and words that sometimes fills my chest, making me dizzy and unable to concentrate. Or forgetting essential things. Or when I do something suddenly and get told off for not thinking. These things I can't explain encroach on my ability to see what I can only imagine my personality actually is.

Claire won't talk to many people, which makes me curious. I talk to everyone because it feels necessary – which horrifies my parents. If someone is lovely, they sort of shine and make my heart hurt – I have to tell them. Claire says people who talk to 'any old body' are 'weird.' So, if we are out together, I smile instead.

Claire seems 'apart' from any of my own struggles. I revere in her what seems impossible in myself. Mum says she is 'enduring,' which fascinates and exhausts me equally. It also makes me think of trees.

My confusion once piqued when Claire said she wanted to be an actress. I had thought, 'But surely, everyone would just see that she was still Claire!' And anyway, why would someone so unmistakable want to pretend to be someone else!?

Dear Reader, may I invite you alongside me to view this childhood experience through a lens of compassion.

Because 'behaviour' mattered most to people, the ADHD traits that made me 'meish' also made it impossible to know myself. Eventually, I took this time, and it wasn't personality I found so much as a sense of who I am beyond the traits I once defined myself by. Journaling is still the vessel that brings me back to myself; mindfulness is like magic.

It seems unfair that passive traits like 'not listening,' 'forgetting,' 'clumsiness' or 'overwhelm' became misconstrued as intentional behaviours when the gap in understanding around ADHD was filled with fear. And I feel compassion for anyone feeling 'demonised' as a child for these reasons. When associative triggers arise (from having been seen as 'wrong' before I could even understand what that meant), it means that doing anything wrong, even as an adult, revives that shame. Due to ongoing bloopers, this is where my work towards self-compassion is still going strong.

Anyone whose way of being truly resonates with mine, like their seeming discombobulated or knocking stuff over in a shop, fills my heart with tenderness. Finding self-compassionate makes us more compassionate, a phenomenon that studies by Kristin Neff support.

A Beacon of Hope

'There is a wise being living inside of you. It is your intuitive self. Focus your awareness into a deep place in your body, a place where your 'gut feelings' reside.' – Shakti Gawain.

1982

Deciding on subject options sent me into a spin. History, Childcare, Environmental Study. Supposedly, I'd been learning these subjects, but now they all just look like words. I always have to wait for 'the feeling' to happen, because it's the only way to know things. But nothing comes. The guidelines say to choose subjects that go together in a useful combination for the career I want to pursue. But the only professions I know about are teaching, nursing, and social work, and they need maths. I wonder about myself and can't find a place inside myself from which to make this decision.

Four weeks into the summer holiday, after sitting exams, I didn't even see coming, I read in the library about a nearby sixth-form college offering subjects called psychology and sociology. Something about the nature of inquiry within these subjects excites me.

And I'm on it. Filling out the application, arranging the interview, gathering references, planning the train journey, the funding help, and even finding a Saturday job at a toy shop in the college town. I feel like the master of my destiny. The thrill of being 'in process' is terrifying. I can't eat or sleep, but I don't stop until everything is arranged.

On reflection, I see now how these subjects, and their promise of self-understanding and insight into the world, stood out like a beacon of hope.

Dear Reader, may I invite you alongside me to view this childhood experience through a lens of compassion.

Around this time, I realised it was OK to feel scared and uncomfortable if it meant I'd thank myself later. I feel compassion for my younger self, that it required such fear to 'push through.'

It still does, and writing this book is a good example. I know the same old feeling will return when it comes to publishing, and I know to brace myself for it – 'arm myself' with lavender and hot baths, long walks, nutritious food, daytime naps, and, of course, compassion.

Until my thyroid health dipped, I pushed through everything at full throttle (the chemicals released during sustained stress, I learn, probably contributed to the disease). Taking the downtime I needed to heal was excruciating on many levels. When I couldn't push anymore, when I could only manage ten minutes of anything before conking out - I began to question my worth.

On reflection, perhaps the preciousness of being becomes highlighted when our ability to physically or mentally 'do' in our usual way is compromised.

I never did 'get my maths' and I just wish someone had reassured me that life was possible without it.

When the World Offers an Opening

'Your sacred space is wherever you can find yourself over and over again.' – Joseph Campbell.

1982

I wake up in the little Z bed next to my new friend. I feel fresh and light, as though the world has offered me an opening. There is nothing to work out! I wish I could always feel this way. Perhaps painting my bedroom yellow, like this one, would help? The thought of my bedroom, my unfinished things, my... me-ness. I don't want to go home. I spend the entire day holding onto this unencumbered feeling. My parents came to collect me, but I realise that, somehow, I was already collected. The part of me that has found a home in the knowledge that this lightness, this inner space, is possible, steps into the opening and doesn't look back.

Dear Reader, may I invite you alongside me to view this childhood experience through a lens of compassion.

As a child, I kept vigil to particular feelings. So often, these were a 'lightness' or a 'clearness,' believing that if I tried hard enough, it would 'stay.' When it was gone, I experienced disorientation. How does a feeling become lost?! I would feel 'beside myself' in the truest sense, slightly dissociated. I feel self-compassion for the disappointment that came with my mind wafting from clarity back into ADHD chaos again.

Clarity can be elusive and slow to arrive. 'But', as I reassure my younger self, 'it does come.'

Still Confused

'If we can share our story with someone who responds with empathy and understanding, shame can't survive.' – Brené Brown.

1983

My feelings fill the whole room. Embarrassed at how vast I am, I blame my body for letting it show. The cycle I thought would never begin brings up the rejection of my whole being and rage that leaves me shaking. I bellow because I am scared, uncomfortable, and confused. My access to joy and creativity is suddenly unreliable.

Dear Reader, may I invite you alongside me to view this childhood experience through a lens of compassion.

Spending your life feeling guilty about doing things you didn't understand your reasons for doing makes for a heavy load.

Distinguishing shame from guilt highlighted

my confusion. Using the above example, my initial shame (about my way of being) preceded my guilt feelings (that I upset people by shouting). As an adult with ADHD, I feel some self-compassion knowing that my first response to shame was to feel shame for feeling it – let's not go there!

Perhaps we can recognise there is nothing shameful about feeling shame, especially when we have just stepped out of our confusion and realise that – up until now – our bag labelled shame, inside our bag labelled guilt, has been sealed in a bag marked 'confusion.'

So often, our intention is just to understand ourselves or to be understood. But before we get the answers to our confusion, how can we know that the hidden, pulsing beat of shame cannot survive for long in the light of the truth about our neurology?

Peculiar Landscape

'I think I can tell the wrong sort for myself thanks'
– JK Rowling, The Philosopher's Stone.

1983

It would be a long time before I could tell the 'wrong sort' for myself. Aged nearly fifteen, the secondary school newbie, I have allowed myself to be 'snapped up' by whoever will have me and feel a keen sense of danger. Increasingly, I feel in the wrong body, house, town, and school with the wrong friends. I'm trying to make sense of this peculiar landscape, but despite my heavy kicker boots, the effort to stay upright suggests an adverse camber.

Immediately pegged as spacey, my new peers wave a hand in front of me and say 'heeeellllllooo.' A teacher asks me sarcastically if I have left myself at home. I answer literally: 'Yes, I think so.' My exit from the classroom earns me kudos I neither want nor deserve. My chaos catches others around me in my net.

Dear Reader, may I invite you alongside me to view this childhood experience through a lens of compassion.

When I read this back, the overwhelm of too much change (including hormonal) leaps off the page. Or perhaps hormones were the most significant change and, too often, the afterthought.

I keenly feel compassion for all girls from 'generation shame' around periods. Hormones exacerbate ADHD symptoms, and I feel sad that it took until menopause for questions about ADHD to arise.

I wonder how many more women with ADHD have to reach this life change to believe they are seriously losing it to anxiety or forgetfulness. I feel compassion for us all and realise my concern has unfolded into a flat sheet and become one of the purposes of this book.

A Path to Emotional Regulation

'Music evokes emotion, and emotion can bring its memory.' – Oliver Sacks.

1985

I'm sixteen and beginning to offer my dad my own song discoveries. I'm officially labelled a 'difficult' teenager, yet through sharing music, confusion and difficulty gave way to connection. When he died in a horrible accident, his passing left a gaping hole of silence where music used to be.

Once my path to emotional-regulation, music became pain itself.

The air is thick with unplayed songs. I stop listening to music altogether, daring only to 'play it' in my head. But every now and then, a song I've been carefully preserving in my heart, allowing myself to 'hear' just the opening harmony of, perhaps – plays disrespectfully, without warning in a supermarket or gets used for a TV advert, and I sort of collapse inside. So I stopped going into shops and went upstairs during the adverts.

For over two decades, I made no new associations with this music, and in not doing so, the grief it brought up in me was always raw. I became, quite literally, terrified of hearing it.

Dear Reader, may I invite you alongside me to view this childhood experience through a lens of compassion.

For so long, I could only feel sorry that my dad had lost his life. Untimely deaths are confusing, and pain became the new axis around which the family spun. But now, I can feel compassion for my younger self, who (unknowingly), let go of a powerful tool for emotional regulation in an effort to preserve the last link to a parent.

Rough Terrain

'Some things in life cannot be fixed. They can only be carried.' – Megan Devine.

1985

The inner world of loss was a new landscape to navigate, and returning to college after my dad's passing felt like crossing rough terrain. It took a while to realise that the college hadn't been informed. I had started to think that perhaps it wasn't so big of a deal, that people's parents probably die all the time, and that I should just be 'getting on with it.' But I couldn't seem to get to classes. I wandered the town through the strange, thick air. I spent a lot of time staring. A childhood friend later told me that I wrote to her–reams of thoughts and feelings.

At college, my absences eventually culminated in an angry outburst by a tutor, and I remember running between the desks shouting, 'Why is everything just carrying on? Don't you know my dad died?!' But something about studying felt safe, and I let it absorb me.

Mum wasn't 'herself' for a while, but many years later, we shared the understanding that there just didn't seem to be anyone there for a time. But then, somehow, my parent's oldest, dearest friends gathered us up.

Dear Reader, may I invite you alongside me to view this young adult experience through a lens of compassion.

Remembering how we flailed, I can still feel the incredulity of my younger self, experiencing the intense insult that was breakfast TV on the morning following my dad's death. I can now find self-compassion that, at the edge of my awareness, sat the belief that being a 'difficult teenager' had contributed wholeheartedly to this tragedy.

We all need coping strategies, and knowing what they are can be the first step to using them autonomously. In retrospect, hyper-focusing on a project was my coping strategy. I found peace in the gentle forward motion of writing. This way of dealing with grief repeats itself.

Eight isn't a Value; It's a Shape.

'...harness individual interests and abilities to inform and transform approaches to daunting situations.' – Renee Hamilton-Newman.

1988

I work for a building society as a cashier.

'Well, he didn't employ her for her maths skills, did he!' scoffs a colleague from the faraway land of the capable, directly behind me.

I'm desperately trying to work out how £1000 has 'gone missing' from my till. How do I even begin? I'm told that because of the amount, this might need to be a police matter. But my brain won't work. Even the numbers themselves don't make sense anymore. Eight stops being a value and becomes a shape again, the joined-up snake of primary school. As the manager leans over me too closely, I fade in and out.

I'm hit by a wave of confusion, 'Why did I

go for this job? I ask myself, remembering the thrill of applying for something beyond my capability.

The manager explains that I put £1000 too much into my computer this morning, so I'm £1000 down this evening. His voice doesn't sound reassuring, and I can see smirking faces and angry glances. I've held everyone up tonight.

On the bus home, in the exercise book I keep with me, I write it all out, hoping that if I write slowly, missing nothing out, I will comprehend in a way I can't in a 'live' situation. I write:

'When I cashed up this evening, there was £1000 less money. It said I had £4900 cash on my screen and in my till, I had £3900. £4900 take away £3900 is £1000 difference. Hooray, because this is the amount of money missing. So how did this happen? I must have lost £1000 in cash or put £1000 too much into the system this morning. The £1000 was missing on the computer at sign-off because I must have put in £1000 more than my usual £2400 at sign-on, but it never was cash in my till. So it's not actually missing. It's just what the computer says should be in the till at sign-off. This is true because we looked at my sign-in sheet, which was £3400'.

Understood.

Dear Reader, may I invite you alongside me to view this experience through a lens of compassion.

Why on earth did I work at a Building Society?! If I could do what I was most unable to - maths - which made me constantly feel inadequate, I wouldn't be!

I feel compassion for my younger self, who thought it was necessary to put myself into situations that proved my limits rather than demonstrating my capabilities.

Learning to respect our limits, gives us the freedom to work right up to their edges, which can turn out to be greater freedom than we imagine.

Calm in a Crisis

'Perhaps it's the innate hyper-focus. Or the adrenaline rush. Or the years we've spent working hard to ignore buzzing, beeping, unimportant distractions. For maybe all of these reasons, and many others, ADHD brains tend to shine in times of emergency.' – The Editorial Board of ADDitude.

1990

As a young first-time parent, I experienced motherhood as an ongoing emergency. Aged just twenty and still reeling at the loss of my dad, the utter love, fear, and demands that came with being a mum kept me on high alert for years.

'So,' I conclude. My struggles have just been selfishness, laziness, carelessness, and immaturity. I was an awful person, and it seems parenting is the making of me!

The various calamities that might have sent me into a spin before were now par for the course. But over time, the boys' growing capabilities reduced my urgency, and 'it' started again.

I have been that 'ditsy mum' in their eyes ever since, yet I'm still the first person my kids call in a crisis.

Dear Reader, may I invite you alongside me to view this experience through a lens of compassion.

I parented my boys up in 'crisis mode' - there was so much fear around being a parent, and the tenuous nature of life had become part of my understanding.

Unwittingly, the adrenaline constantly pumping through my body made me a walking reaction. It masked my ADHD, and at times, made me feel super-capable. I feel compassion for the confusion that arose when the crisis went into a lull, and my struggles with executive function reappeared tenfold.

In retrospect, as a child, I sometimes created the sort of crisis that adversely affected others, and I couldn't understand why it was so relieving! Maybe we still scare ourselves by doing things 'off the cuff,' but as adults, we can begin to trust our ethics and values to guide us.

Over Doing (and Under Being)

'Nature does not hurry, and yet everything is accomplished.' – Lao Tzu.

1992

When my boys were little, I renamed my approach to life 'multitasking.' My variable attention came into its own, the demands of being a parent offering endless opportunities to be 'creative in the moment.' I was hyperactive 24/7, relentlessly trying to 'get there.' And 'there' meant being prepared for tomorrow.

I'm twenty-three. Being a parent is a serious business, and I hold myself to working a 'day ahead.' I can no longer afford to notice my feelings about my undone things or my way of thinking and being in the world. I nurture active scorn around my childhood struggles and call it 'all that kid stuff.'

My oldest son's ADHD went undiagnosed until his late teens. I had assumed all six-year-olds needed to be taken out for a jog in the evening.

My brain feels a different shape in the world. I don't keep getting 'stuck' – but have lots of accidents and near-misses and secretly fear these prove I am not a capable parent. So, I keep working a day ahead to prove I am.

But while in the throes of over-doing and under-being, I lost my connection to my essential nature. I missed the signs of unhealthy relationships and became busy making pleasing people an end in itself.

Dear Reader, may I invite you alongside me to view this childhood experience through a lens of compassion.

Reflecting, I can see how my ADHD 'differences' played out over decades and decades of scenarios. Questions like – 'Who's that (very famous) person? And 'What do you mean the 'lol' my sons put at the end of their texts means laugh out loud? (It means lots of love, doesn't it?) - tell me I am always one step behind.

Scooby and Shaggy's legs in a perfect circular blur come to mind when I read this last paragraph. They run with all their might only to realise that they have gotten nowhere, that the monster is holding the backs of their collar and T-shirt, respectively. In expending so much energy on 'flight,' little is left to 'fight' with. Maybe, though, the shape of a fight can become different in the light of new understandings rather than raising awareness, rather than self-defence.

I can find compassion around my inability to hold the truth of my being up to the light. In dismissing my childhood feelings, I invalidated myself. I wasn't 'suddenly an adult'; I was a full-time over-compensator.

When it came to my boys, I struggled with emotional regulation. The love I felt was frequently overwhelming, its intensity tangled with the grief of losing my dad. I was fiercely protective, probably displacing the fight I might have more evenly distributed among all my relationships. My now-adult sons rib me with their memories of my legging it across playgrounds or parks, chasing approval and feeling the need to 'give people verbal' on their behalf.

Maybe, in our own ways, we all seek external validation from strangers in the park. Perhaps what matters most is to recognise we are doing it.

The Huge Wordless Question

'In contradiction and paradox, you can
find truth.' – Denis Villeneuve.

1993

I am a young mum at twenty-four years old.
It's a Thursday, and my boys, aged four and
five, are at school.

'What do you mean you feel like a
contradiction!?' Jenni's voice rises to the
ceiling. 'You can't feel like that!' she
demands. 'Look at your life. You've got so
many youish things going on.'

The bright emerald kitchen tiles draw
me from our eye contact over and over,
threatening to transport me into that weird
vacant place, and the itchiness of my
vest top label flickers in and out of my
consciousness. The radio is on low, but
my ear picks out every other word – so
I only hear fragments of what Jenni says.
Our conversation is disjointed, and I keep
saying, 'Sorry?' Meanwhile, in my peripheral

vision, the titles of cookery books entice me until I feel compelled to rise mid-sentence and check them out. Youish. A word that holds equal condemnation as praise.

My mother's wail of 'Do you always have to be so youish?!' juxtaposed with her sincerest, 'Wow, that's a great idea, song, poem, picture darling - it's just so youish,' creating bewilderment in me then, resurfaces now, catching me off guard.

'Well, I do feel like that,' I mutter incoherently from a suspended place. 'I always have.' But Jenni is a 'school mum friend,' and any minute now, her kindly enquiring expression will transform into the kindly but baffled one I usually encounter.

The cookery books are nondescript. My head begins to fuzz as I cross the threshold of social engagement and into the realm of 'ordeal.' I have dared to express a feeling about myself and have been told I can't feel it. Excusing myself in a familiar burst of 'must,' I sit on the stone floor of the bathroom with a thud of knowing. I am alone with this deep confusion about my confusion. 'I'll get there' comes my predictable return. Lately, though, part of me is unsure where 'there' is.

The huge wordless question weaves relentlessly through my experience. The once vague strands – thinly delivered comments, gather into echoing remarks and form knots. In my only way of working things out – to trust that when the answer came, I would 'hear' it, I cradle my untidy tangle and wait for an end to appear.

Dear Reader, may I invite you alongside me to view this childhood experience through a lens of compassion.

In this ordinary situation, I was experiencing ADHD overwhelm. Zoning out of the present moment due to sensory and emotional overload, I begin operating from a 'suspended place,' all the while struggling to interact 'normally.' Unwittingly, my girlfriend invalidated my experience by exclaiming, 'You can't feel like that!' and proffered a word that triggered further confusion.

Before learning about my neurology, I did feel like a contradiction. I still do, to some extent, feel confused about my capabilities. So often, something I know should be easy ends up impossible, and something seemingly impossible seems easy. How can I pull together a singing performance but ask me to set a dinner table, and I break a sweat!?

I feel compassion for my younger self, who longed to be true to one focus but was trawled by sudden unexpected interests and ideas that fizzed with potential, and then fizzled out entirely.

As adults diagnosed with ADHD, the big wordless question now answered might make us think 'if only.' Perhaps to find self-compassion for our late learning curve, we might be gentle as we process and give ourselves time to adjust to what this new understanding means to us, both now and to our childhood selves.

Green Time

'Look deep into nature, and then you will understand everything better.' – Albert Einstein.

1993

Sometime in my early twenties, three days into workplace training, which had seen me chin prop sleep several times in front of new colleagues, one asked me jokingly if I was narcoleptic. For the facilitator's question, 'Am I boring you?' I have no answer and feel dizzy trying to work it out.

In the break, I decide to go searching for some peace and to ponder the question. Was I bored?   It's bothered me to have appeared rude and unprofessional, and I don't feel able to return. So I take a bus and sit on the grass in the botanical gardens in Cambridge. It's lovely here, and I know why I have come. I need to revisit something that once gave me an indescribable feeling, an absence of complication. Something from before this confused version of myself and before there were so many words in my head. I begin trying to return to my childhood garden. I close my eyes. No. Open them. I need to see the flowers, the colours. I attempt to enter my younger self's mind and look through her eyes. From inside my despair, I attempt a feeling when I look at the bright blue flowers and the vivid green of the grass and instead notice that the word vert suits green more than the word green does. I began regretting that I could never learn French properly and that, like most things, it eventually became too complicated. It takes a while before I realise my mind has drifted, that I am still just myself with all my chaos, trying.

It must be just a memory. A memory of an indescribable feeling I know might be forever lost.

Dear Reader, may I invite you alongside me to view this childhood experience through a lens of compassion.

I trust nature's chaos in ways I can't extend to myself. But I know now why I enjoy its guilt-free mess: it's variable enough to hold my attention and regulates chaos in its invisibly perfect, unique cycle.

Although the workshop's subject wasn't interesting, I believed I should be able to sustain interest. Nowadays, I'm suspicious of 'shoulds' because they are usually someone else's agenda, a societal 'norm,' and don't accommodate my neurology.

We can only optimise our optimum way of working when it's on our radar. So, in the light of having ADHD, instead of asking ourselves, 'Can we be bored and hide it?' Perhaps the question becomes, 'How can we purposefully cope with boredom?'

To Be as I Am

'Since your ADD can't be cured, your goal shouldn't be to eliminate your deficits. Instead, it should be to identify, accept and manage them.' – Kate Kelly and Peggy Ramundo.

1993

At many of life's junctures, given that my sense of time is so 'loopy' I have hankered after the feeling of who I was before self-consciousness. That this book began in my childhood garden is, I realise, no accident. The place I started is the place I yearn to return to – to presence, un-selfconsciousness, and life untouched by feelings of 'difference.' Sometimes, my memory of this feeling feels so close I could almost reach out and touch it.

According to authors Kelly and Ramundo, making the self-assessment that you are not lazy, crazy, or stupid is 'central to your recovery.' Without an ADHD diagnosis, these are precisely the assumptions that can become our truths, leaving nothing to identify, accept, and manage.

A process of 'eliminating' the undesirable parts of myself began early, manifesting in trying very hard at things I could never be good at, and feeling no sense of achievement or worth around what I could do well.

As a young mum, I had a keen sense that the people around me felt that I needed 'putting right' somehow. It was open season on my way of doing and being. Various responses to my vegetarianism, poetry, mural painting, vintage clothes, studying, and homemade baby food all seemed to culminate in a shared rating: 'not normal' -aka, unacceptable. Among other young mums, I felt 'apart from', not part of, their community. A curiosity to occasionally invite in, make a point that they haven't got any of my 'funny tea bags' - only 'normal ones' - and to interrogate.

Then, one bright sunny day, while on the cusp of losing touch with myself completely, I assisted an old friend with his ancestry search. Following some energetic ivy ripping, we found the grave of his great-great-grandfather. I remember thinking, 'Hidden in our forebears' lives are clues to ourselves.' I felt wistful, hoping mine had felt allowed to be who they were and felt accepted and cherished. It then hit me that I wanted this for my children – for them to be who they are wholeheartedly.

Then I thought of my children, born into the world such whole little beings. Might they one day be subjected to the scrutiny of others and find themselves lacking? A maternal blast of pain seared through me for their pain. But something else emerged too: the realisation that it was my birthright to be as I am. When to be 'allowed' this, my deepest need, came into my consciousness; I felt found.

Dear Reader, may I invite you alongside me to view this childhood experience through a lens of compassion.

My tendency to revisit my early memories no longer feeds the belief that I am stupid, lazy, or crazy. And I know now that I can move forward because I am no longer fixated on the past to find answers. Instead, early memories remind me that it's possible for my being to be present.

While walking in nature, I need not be self-conscious; I am in good company, and this feels restorative.

Not So Super-Market

'Organising is what you do before you do something so that when you do it, it's not all mixed up.' – A. A. Milne.

1994

As a young mum, there was only one way to supermarket shop. I do a little reconnaissance work. Pen and paper in hand, I walk up and down, write the aisle numbers, and make headings.

Then I go home and make a list of every food I ever need, cut the list up into items and glue them under the relevant aisles. Voila. Down to the library and a few photocopies later, I have a list tailored to the local supermarket. Each week I tick what I need, and one aspect of life becomes maybe one percent more manageable. This process is an ongoing exercise because otherwise, I experience the inevitable quarterly re-arrangement of shelves as a rewire that's happened inside my brain!

I did try the 'normal' way. Of course, I did. List in hand, my baby and toddler in the trolley, the overwhelm that ensues when looking from list to shelf list to shelf is total. Physically dizzying. Then, confusingly, on other days, I mysteriously embody efficiency.

Dear Reader, may I invite you alongside me to view this childhood experience through a lens of compassion.

A live supermarket shop is still challenging. I feel compassionate towards the 'ridiculous but necessary efforts' of my younger self and want to whisper to her that one day, something called online shopping will raise this aspect of life to around ten percent more manageable.

There are many examples of 'ridiculous but necessary effort' in this book, and I use the word ridiculous here to mean highly incongruous. In the example used, I found it monumentally difficult that facing a task that looked easy for everyone else required the same diligence as essay writing. That simply didn't make sense.

Being told 'you are making it difficult for yourself' was a phrase I had heard often and interpreted as meaning I was subconsciously doing this on purpose.

I now aim to meet such confusion with self-compassion. To gently reframe my 'ways of doing' as acceptable, creative and downright courageous! We live in a society that assumes fully functioning executive functions. We might begin to wonder whether what is truly ridiculous is not ourselves - but that very assumption.

Wodge

'Normal is just a cycle on a washing machine.'
– Whoopi Goldberg.

2000

I remember asking my good friend what he was doing one morning; it was a beautiful day. Did he want to go out? He said he was doing his washing. I laughed and said it sounded like the excuse, 'not tonight, I'm washing my hair,' but he was earnest. I couldn't believe he thought clothes washing was something you 'do.'

'How else will it get done?' he asks.

I think of the washing that sits in the machine for days until I notice it, or the garments that get rained on and dried au naturel later in the week.

'You just make excuses so you don't have to do it properly,' he says.

And I wonder if I'm lazy - because everything's a bit like that.

Dear Reader, may I invite you alongside me to view this childhood experience through a lens of compassion.

It occurs to me now to write out all the steps that make up 'doing the laundry' from beginning to end. Not exactly riveting stuff, but please hang in there (pardon the pun):

Sort clothes from the hamper and take them downstairs (without getting distracted by anything else)

Put the wash on.

Get washing out (if you remember to)

Hang out on the line

Take down (if you remember that it's hanging out)

Give it a five-minute tumble and:

Get it out (if you haven't already wandered off)

Take upstairs for sorting

Sort some (that's never going to happen in one go)

Put away sorted items.

So, there are ten steps and four possible distraction points (the significant time required between each step). There is a reason I struggle with this task, and having a reason is not the same as making an excuse.

Underneath It All

'Everybody is a genius, but if you judge a fish by its ability to climb a tree, it will live its whole life believing it is stupid.' – Albert Einstein.

2001

I'm in my early thirties, working in a gift shop. It's nearly Christmas. The concentration it takes to check off stock numbers correctly this morning, while the shop bustles with Saturday customers has made my head fuzzy. Numbers tend to turn themselves into other numbers. The new stock makes me stare. Hand-made, embroidered purses, tiny notebooks, gemstones, and silk scarves transport me. Somewhere warm and colourful is where I keep slipping away to.

Feeling embarrassed having to ask my colleague to repeat an instruction yet again because I had listened but not 'heard,' I remark that I am having a 'dippy day' today. Her return scoff to a customer of, 'Dippy life more like,' fills my throat with aching thickness, adding weight to the 'keep ups' and 'don't you get it's' which had spattered my school years. She says I make her uncomfortable in her next breath because she feels that 'underneath it all,' I'm clever. It was an accusation, and I wondered if she was waiting for some sort of confession.

Speechless for a moment, the constriction in my throat feels self-inflicted. I have caught a glimpse of how I am seen.

On reflection, I might have been flattered that someone thought I could have the confidence and ability to fake being 'dippy.' Had I made her feel fooled?

Escaping tears and betray my sensitivity. And after phoning in sick a couple of times, it feels necessary – not for the first time - to leave a nice little job because of feeling I had been exposed as not enough. I won't walk past the shop. I will wonder for ages about the 'underneath it all' my colleague had referred to.

Dear Reader, may I invite you alongside me to view this childhood experience through a lens of compassion.

I have finally understood my 'dippyness' to be what people see at the juncture where my executive functions struggle with something I have absolutely no interest in, where I zone out through boredom. But this has nothing to do with intelligence, and everything to do with saving myself for what sparks me and giving it my best shot.

My self-esteem dropped a notch following this exchange, and I feel compassion for my younger self that I had no understanding to 'come back with' when people said things like this, and instead internalised their words as truth.

I still struggle when I hear people talk about someone in terms of their being, as 'the sort of person who never finishes anything' or 'the sort of person who can't stick at a job.' It makes me scream inside. It makes me want to write a book about the lived experience of ADHD!

A Something Else

'It's worrying, Katy, that you are a really bad dancer, but so confident with it.' – An honest friend.

2002

I write L and R on my hands and put stickers on my shoes, but still flounder at the merest instruction. My dancing classes, hilarious as they are humiliating, are excellently delivered.

I must work out every movement and hope the lag doesn't show. I have to remember which leg and arm is which, over and over, and can't rely on natural rhythm to guide me.

Dear Reader, may I invite you alongside me to view this childhood experience through a lens of compassion.

I wouldn't necessarily have put struggles with spatial awareness in the category of something that mattered, until having those classes. Bumping into people and objects was just my normal.

Dancing required a 'something else,' and I feel compassion that trying to fathom what, led me down a confidence eroding path. I couldn't understand, because I loved to dance free style, yet a sequence of a few steps in a class was a mental and physical struggle to hold. There was nowhere to hide my difficulty on a dance floor, and I left under a cloud of the same wan excuses I used for my brief attempts at Karate, Street Dance, Tai Chi, and yoga. Dyspraxia, a neurodevelopmental condition linked to ADHD, didn't occur. Already labelled 'clumsy,' I thought I just had to try harder!

It's not unusual to believe we just have to 'try harder' before we know we are neurodivergent. The action of trying harder because we feel we are lacking is called overcompensating. Recognising what we struggle with can soothe our anxiety, allowing us to access our creativity and 'try differently', rather than harder.

Unfriending

'Friendship with oneself is all important, because without it one cannot be friends with anyone else in the world.' – Eleanor Roosevelt.

2003

Aged just fifty-four, my beautiful, terminally ill mum makes her way through the cards friends have sent her. It seems she needs to express her particular grievance with each. 'I can now,' she says, 'because it is the end.' She harks back to a woman she lent a knitting pattern to in the seventies, then had returned only a photocopy. A 'friend' who ignored her arthritis, taking her on a rocky walk and going on about her own robust joints. And people whose jealousy about aspects of my mum's easy nature led them to say cruel things.

'I don't suppose they are jealous now,' she says.

Witnessing this one-sided showdown was a powerful turning point for my relationships.

My horror at the thought of having to 'wait until the end' to be true to myself sent me on a bit of an 'un-friender bender' before unfriending was even a thing.

Dear Reader, may I invite you alongside me to view this childhood experience through a lens of compassion.

I think about this a lot lately. Life is fleeting. Approaching fifty-four myself, I begin to 'take stock', as my mum might have, had she known her time on earth was limited. Real friends share your fleeting achievements and joys, recognizing that success is just when something aligns for a while.

Sometimes I think narcissistic people can sniff out ADHDers from across a room. Lately, having been stung many times and hooked into being 'used,' I try to spot them first!

Being authentic may always be met with a raised eyebrow, but never by real friends. I feel compassion for my mum and for myself at our untimely parting and believe that a life lived is a whole life, however short or long.

We may spend a lifetime learning ways to comfortably assert our feelings to other people about their behaviour. But maybe what matters first, and most, is learning to listen to those feelings and to become completely congruent with ourselves.

New Life

'Sometimes when you're in a dark place you think you've been buried, but you've actually been planted.' – Christine Caine.

2004

To my great delight, I am a new mum again at thirty-five! The natural demands of motherhood begin where caring for my mum ended. In this relentless response mode, I am twenty again and can busy away my grief by 'doing.' I finish my degree, take on a part-time project co-ordinating job – a Time Bank, wherein everyone's abilities are viewed equally – and secretly work full-time hours because everything I do on the computer takes so long. My newsletters are cut and pasted (literally), and even though I have a diary, there seems to be no way to remember things! What's wrong with me? I begin wondering why being a stay-at-home Mum is so hard, then realise I can't run a household either! One morning, I can't even coordinate a cup of tea; I call it a 'breakdown'. Nothing makes sense – maybe grief finally caught up.

Dear Reader, may I invite you alongside me to view this experience through a lens of compassion.

My struggles with executive function had revealed themselves. This was an ADHD shutdown and while it was happening, I truly believed my brain would never recover. It was frightening, I couldn't talk or think properly, and I clung to my dog for dear life, not wanting my 'brokenness' to affect my daughter.

There have been physical health consequences for my years of being a human 'doing' – entirely out of touch with my 'beingness.' I can feel self-compassion for those particularly dynamic and super-duper strivings that served my neurology but ultimately may have contributed to my auto-immune thyroid condition.

I reflect, too, with curiosity around my ADHD inheritance - that my dad, a fireman, had been a first responder. 'Expecting the bleeper' had been an everyday part of our family life.

Whatever way we 'expect the bleeper,' in

our lives, learning to prepare for it in the light of our neurodivergence is self-compassionate.

Part Three:
Talking to a Pie About
Walking the Dog

Nevertheless, Bliss

'Kindred spirits are not so scarce as I used to think. It's splendid to find out there are so many of them in the world.' — L.M. Montgomery, Anne of Green Gables.

2005

A soundscape of pings and chimes accompanies the soft voice guiding me to bring my awareness to my feet. I ponder on the sounds. The chimes seem to stun me, and I lose the next instruction. I'm still on my feet. The voice asks me to move my awareness to my knees. I wonder if it's OK that I missed my calves. I attempt to tune into myself and 'the breath' and fall asleep, not quite the idea, I know, but nevertheless blissful!

I felt immediately accommodated walking into this beautiful Quaker building for an absolute, treat-to-self week of mindful meditation.

There's a low hum in my head now. My heart aches contemplating the decades of thoughts and prayers that have permeated these wood-panelled walls; I add my own.

Midweek, I manage to dare a little. Dare to look at the nature of my mind. It feels like an otherworldly experience, this being welcomed to be myself–gratitude wells in me as I recognise that I am among kindred souls here. We talk about what it means to be human, to bring our whole selves to our work as teachers, therapists, writers, parents and carers. We learn what it means to be genuinely congruent, and practice it there in the room. I can sense the 'edginess' of this work, that we are each at varying degrees of tilt. I feel my angle keenly. But it's OK; this is a safe space, a haven. Being here is all there is because there's nothing to pull me away. There is no 'something else I need to do' for once. Even in my head! Wandering mind…. back to 'the breath.' Wandering mind… back to 'the breath.' Here, I can meet the challenge of noticing what happens when I am experiencing, without the struggle between my mind, body and soul that so often feels part of who I am. In the absence of the confusion that everyday life presents, I 'come together' here and wish, beg, pray –all of those -to learn how I might, on an ordinary day, more easily access this way of being. This... dimension of present moment awareness.

I have come here to find ways to help me relax. Is it paradoxical that I have come here to find ways to 'help me down,' but that finding I can relax makes me feel over-excited? Maybe I'm wasting my time?

By late afternoon on the fourth day, I experienced something 'switch' in my head during the guided meditations. The practice enables a stillness that doesn't 'suck me in' as does a book or an interest. Nor do I drift into a familiar fuzzy mindspace. Perhaps I am, in the facilitator's words, 'cultivating alertness' by noticing my thoughts and naming their type 'An Idea', 'a Worry,' a Fantasy, Wishful Thinking or Looking for Certainty. This, rather than suppressing them, engaging with them, judging them, reacting to them or creating a narrative. This is a brand new 'something to do'!

Experiencing my thoughts this way offers me new possibilities for living inside myself. Surely now I can decide whether to drift into 'staring mode,' or stop losing days to a single activity?

But recently, alarmingly, even my sense of that experience has felt tenuous. I haven't 'practised.' For ten days, my home practice was keen and robust, punctuated by short meditations but familiarly, it dwindled until ceasing entirely. And while I can hear it calling now, it's as though I can't 'tune in.'

Dear Reader, may I invite you alongside me to view this experience through a lens of compassion.

I recognise this encounter with my mind's way filled me with hope. Perhaps I can find some compassion that I missed the point by striving to 'store the moment for future reference,' while at the same time trying to experience it! By entering the moment and looking at its true nature, I might have noticed that it passes and passes and passes, and that attempting to store a moment as more than memory was borne of desperation.

I see now that a blissful state is more accessible in an environment conducive to relaxation than in 'the world.' Being 'guided' meant not needing to rely on my own motivation. Perhaps I might not choose to further diminish myself with a barrage of unkind words. In the spirit of mindful self-compassion, I wonder if I can offer myself the possibility that it's acceptable that my practice waned. Life is busy. I am buoyed by learning that remembering to 'come back to the breath' is the practice that strengthens the neural pathway that brings more mindful moments into our lives.

I am human, have ADHD neurology, and, without a reminder, will forget to 'notice my breath.' So I appreciate that it keeps going and trust that random mindful moments are as helpful as planned ones.

As adults with ADHD, when something feels new again – enough to be stimulating, we might find joy in having another go. To take from it what we need, relax our goals around it and to practice letting things be what they are for as long as they are.

We may wear many masks in our attempts to 'fit in.' When we begin to recognise this, we become more congruent human beings. Congruence cultivates authenticity, and freedom from the need to wear a 'mask' may be the bliss we seek.

Talking to a Pie About Walking the Dog

'There's no harm in talking to yourself, but try
to avoid telling yourself jokes you've
heard before.' – Ashleigh Brilliant.

2008

Once, when I tried to give up lists and sticky notes.

'Are you talking to me?', my partner sounds irritated.

I say, 'no' for the third time.

'Do you realise you're running a commentary about everything you are doing?'

I hadn't, but it seems that in giving up post-it notes, my need to find a different way to plan had recently manifested in telling myself aloud what I will be doing next. I talk to my washing up about doing the garden, telling it I must put my daughter's school uniform in the wash first. There are lots of 'Rights.' and 'That's that' going on - which I suppose are the equivalent of the resolute peeling off and screwing up of a post-it. Then there are lots of 'Nows' and huffing and frowning followed by 'a ha's.' I run a little in head sketch... 'and she's coming up to the cupboard and opening it and yes! She's found the flour and the butter, and it's coming up to the finish line...... And she's forgotten she was going to do something else entirely.' I glance at the lead on the table avoiding woeful eyes of my beloved Collie, Badger, beneath.

I begin, mindfully as possible as I often do when I start a task. Everything set out; weighed in too many bowls. I breadcrumb gently and move into 'the zone.' Either it's this way of cooking, or it's the 'caffeinated' way that seems to happen even without caffeine! A 'speed of light' 'on pain of death' multitasks relying wholly on the prowess of my hunter-gathering instincts in the kitchen cupboard, resulting in something that always tastes the same because I can't resist putting everything in.

'...Then put my shoes on....' I say.

'Are you talking to me?' My partner calls again. And I catch myself in the moment.

'No. I'd use your name if I were talking to you.' I turn the pastry, start to say something else aloud and then stop. And smile, because I realise, I'm talking to a pie about walking the dog.

Dear Reader, may I invite you alongside me to view this experience through a lens of compassion.

I feel self-compassion when I think of the many times I hated myself for getting over excited and came away from a situation believing I was unacceptable. Even now, I love and hate it equally and have begun trying to just notice it as part of my way. I call it soaring, instead of over-excited. This feels kinder because there's no implicit measurement of my way of being.

I'm not sure I need to find self-compassion around having found a way that works! But I expect people might find compassion for me when they see me talking aloud to myself, though – so perhaps I can leave that one to them.

Priorities

'I know I can either do housework
or have a life.' – Molly B.

2010

My dear friend Molly who – I notice – arms herself with love, humour and music to face the challenges of MS, says with complete certainty that she knows she can either do housework or have a life.

Molly's approach is poignant to me, as it is between housework and life that I often feel 'stuck'. Seeing her decision-making in action looks so brave and free. The distinction my friend seems able to make between what is and what is not worth doing fills me with curiosity. Bothered as to why I haven't got this 'equipment,' I realise that I can't prioritise, and everything seems as essential as everything else.

I am hyper, and my brain is clenched, fizzing with ideas following a particularly sociable morning with members and volunteers at the beloved club Molly runs, and to which she consistently devotes a portion of her heart.

I suspect Molly knows something I don't as she uncurls my hands, that are tight in fists, in sympathy, takes my shoulders, sits me down and tells me to 'just listen' to a piece of music 'and see what happens.' Is my inner world so obvious? I am desperate to appreciate this intervention now. But I can't, and know that, as usual, it will have to be the retrospective version.

I try to fathom her technique, her ability to decide, stop, accept and let be – which are just some of her qualities – but my brain won't go there. I tell myself I'm lacking. Molly seems to know this and tells me kindly not to beat myself up, and that I make up for it in other areas. I'm sorry I never asked her what she meant.

Dear Reader, may I invite you alongside me to view this experience through a lens of compassion.

I wonder if it's possible to pay compassion forward – to yourself? After all, the person being kind to you wants you to experience their kindness. But what about when the most you can do is cope with getting through the moment?

When we are working so hard on the inside to manage our neurology, getting into the 'right space' to gracefully receive kindness in the moment it's offered can seem impossible.

As adults with ADHD, might we later, in another mind space, take time to purposefully reflect on and accept that kindness, let a tremendous loving energy which was meant for us sometime earlier in the day, the month, the year – but that couldn't quite reach – soak in.

An Alternative Way to be Heard

'Drink your tea slowly and reverently, as if it
is the axis on which the world earth revolves –
slowly, evenly, without rushing toward the future;
live the actual moment. Only this moment is life.'
– Thich Nhat Hanh.

Continuing to hum, to warm up, I prepare consciously, dress slowly in a particular order, my mind and body moving into a strange calm. I tell myself there is no need for nerves because I am only getting a dress out of my wardrobe right now. 'I am only putting on shoes…. not on stage until I am. I am only rolling my hair, having a cup of tea, putting on my coat…. not on stage until I am….'

A decade ago, around forty, I became self-employed. What freedom that brought! My partner, a guitarist, had just left his band, and we decided to work together. He created and produced backing tracks and I sang. Beginning first with war songs, we moved into swing jazz, then rockabilly and eventually, I began to think about trying some of the music I loved, dreaded, and missed in equal measure.

When the music starts, I trust I can 'perform'. I always sing a new song at each gig. I can never work out if this is brave or stupid, but I love it! I seem to need to challenge myself, to dare.

The expressive aspect of this work is a way to be heard that isn't responded to with quizzical eyes or an expression akin to amused pity. Many of the songs I sing have been my emotional nemeses, the kind that can wrench me inside with the emotions they evoke, the loved ones they remind me of, and that can shatter me in an instant. But I seem to have found a way to meet them head-on. I sing them out, and their power to cause me pain dissolves. Every note is my most honed tribute to the last and dedication to the next.

New memories are created around these songs, and they no longer 'catch me out' emotionally. Audiences in local pubs and social clubs love the eclectic mix. I am capable, and this doesn't paralyse me like being asked to lay a dinner table does.

Dear Reader, may I invite you alongside me to view this experience through a lens of compassion.

This was an intense time, and I can find compassion for the part of me that didn't understand that it was a healing process - or why she felt she had to 'keep going.' Writing is another way to express myself. It's far more comfortable without an audience, and I don't have to shave my legs! Singing those songs still feels less painful than listening. Maybe because I still don't know where to 'put them.'

Lately, I find myself returning to a childhood love of writing poems, woodland walking, reading and being with dogs – resisting this feels futile!

Maybe part of us instinctively knows what works, even if we always feel on our way to recognising why.

Gently untangling 'how we are' from 'how we think we should be' can be a self-compassionate exercise, and minefield of 'Ah ha' moments. Best tread carefully. Joining an online peer support group and hearing how other neurodivergent people 'do life' can be tremendously validating.

Circles of Time

'Time is not a linear flow, as we think it is, into past, present, and future. Time is an indivisible whole. A great pool in which all events are eternally embodied and still have their meaningful flash of supernormal or extrasensory perception and a glimpse of something that happened long ago in our linear time.' – Frank Waters.

2011

I am in the first year of my counselling diploma. Asked to create a timeline of our lives, the tutor paints a straight line in the air, and there is a collective nod. But that's not how life is! I feel like I did at school. Everyone seeing things one way and me seeing them another. Because what's past can feel as much in the now as now is, so my timeline doesn't follow a line at all. It's more networky. We each were asked to explain.

'Life doesn't go in a straight line, there isn't chronology as such,' I say. 'What I think I know comes back to me for a second or third time for yet another prod to understand it. And sometimes, on the third go-round, I realise I didn't experience what I needed to because I wasn't there enough the first time.' Five pairs of eyes look concerned. Three look down, and one other student cries 'Yes!'

My childhood fascination with time travel becomes clear, my love of books that are not linear but written in the kind of loops that I describe, are all perfect examples of my having to 'come round again' to properly understand. A feeling of calm comes over me when I imagine just living the same day over and over again, nothing new happening: no decisions to make or places to be.

This longing has never escaped my curiosity and is satisfied now in the quiet realisation that I've always known, on some level, that as well as differently shaped days, I need a significant number of 'Inny Days.' The Inny Day needs renaming, though. Although it's a great reset, I notice a part of me still laments that I'm doing life 'wrong.'

Dear Reader, may I invite you alongside me to view this experience through a lens of compassion.

Maybe it's always the 'doing' we struggle with the most. Everyone could spend more time being, after all. I feel compassion for the disorientation I felt when my time blindness and varied attention had me going around in circles.

Yet, although this can be our experience, as embodied beings, we do find ourselves living 'linearly' despite this experience. Seasons change, people and places change. Children grow up. These are all proof that in many ways, we 'move along.'

Part of me is fascinated by the idea of a life lived the same way every day, one that offers me the opportunity to move deeper inside my being and cultivate a new appreciation of the familiar. Life with less stuff. Less commitments. But once I get going on this track, it's too easy to reduce it all down to nothing in my head.

Maybe 'finding a balance' is elusive, and while we might continue to try, it is self-compassionate to recognise it as a 'moving goal' that requires constant attention to discovering one of the thousands of life's combinations – often, our most balanced times are only realised in retrospect.

A Friend in Need

'Saying no can be the ultimate self-care.'
– Claudia Black.

2015

'Why can't you just tell her to f**k off?' My twenty-year-old son is a man of few words. I'm telling him a friend is ringing and texting me every minute of the day with a load of her problems.

And I don't know the answer to this, why saying no seems impossible, or why I can't only have who I choose in my life. He seems to sense my head spin, my struggle 'It's not because I'm stupid', I reassure him, while feeling exactly that. It's not the first time he has known me to have had a friend who seems hell-bent on texting me to death.

And I recognised it then. The moment my child saw me as a person in all my vulnerability. I'm not ready, so, in what feels like a tangible shift, I deflect his question and ask why he hasn't texted his brother yet. We swiftly re-adjust roles, so that he is the son, and I am the mum again.

I later pondered on friendship, on what might be my criteria, and realised I didn't have one. Consistently, I have waited to be asked to dance with anyone who would have me and to any tune. Where is my agency?

Dear Reader, may I invite you alongside me to view this childhood experience through a lens of compassion.

I feel self-compassion that I experienced such wretched confusions around friendship. My younger self had little self-worth and didn't have the agency to assert friend preferences. I just felt grateful if someone offered me the acceptance I craved.

All I can say is, we grow and learn. Self-compassion is a funny thing that grows inside us, making it suddenly possible to be on our 'own side.'

Do we choose friends who abuse our vulnerability? Not on purpose. Do we, on some level, realise what's happening? Maybe. I, for one, just hoped I was wrong.

Ch Ch Ch Changes

'Pretty soon now you're gonna get older.'
– David Bowie, Changes.

2016

I loved to sing but realised, as I entered my seventh year as a jobbing singer with a full calendar, that I was exhausting myself on some level and couldn't 'claw back' my energy – however many supplements I took or early nights I had. My daughter was not yet a teen and grandchildren were coming along! I had been studying to be a person-centred counselor since 2011 so although this was a 'next step,' it still strikes me that making this change wasn't a decision. That as per, I had left my body tell me I had overdone it. I asked myself, 'Do you want to be bopping about on stage after age fifty?' An ABBA-esque answer came back 'Yes, if you want only to eat and sleep and sing….'

On reflection, I feel enormously lucky to have found the course I did, singing and studying overlapped for a while. Our counselling 'classroom' was the Quaker building I'd once visited for a meditation week. Its wooden walls and lattice windows felt like old friends, warmly welcoming me back. In my qualifying year, 2017, I resignedly hung up my dancing shoes, and began working as a counsellor.

Dear Reader, may I invite you alongside me to view this experience through a lens of compassion.

Part of me never reconciled the loss of an activity I enjoyed so much. There was a loss of much more besides singing; joy and challenge, involvement in the unique communities of pubs and clubs, dressing up, and of course, an income. Perhaps self-compassion is the missing piece in this reconciliation. I fight – usually with gratitude as my weapon of choice, to separate the beautiful feelings and memories I have about singing from those of loss.

Perhaps opening up to self-compassion requires looking change in the eye, and treating gratitude and grief not as opposites, but as two sides of the same coin, intensely wonderful, and heartbreakingly painful.

In Too Deep

'There is no greater agony than bearing an untold story inside of you.' – Maya Angelou.

2018

Following the completion of a long-term project, I feel familiarly desperate about the mess that seems to have accumulated while I was 'gone.' When my partner spots me rapidly sorting through our cupboards to chuck out. I feel like I have been caught with my hand in the sweet jar. He says 'You're on one, aren't you.' It's not a question. Luckily, he can't hear the motor in my head. So deep into what I'm doing, I notice how tight my face is. I must look crazy, so immediately relax my expression to look less 'driven' and joke, as always, that he'd better hold onto all his stuff. Then, more sincerely, promise not to throw away anything important.

Time falls away as I grab a bin bag and 'dive in' to smooth my mind. I manage to pick up such a pace that it feels as though I'm doing everything all at once, and in a way, I am. I get halfway through the wardrobe, then flag out and begin on the kitchen cupboards instead. Working to exhaustion, almost nothing is safe from my ousting.

I call it my 'reset', something I believe will 'unstick me' and allow me to function again, and while I imagine this behaviour has to do with recently finishing a project, it doesn't explain why I seem to lose myself to it completely, or my haphazard approach. On no occasion does the space created feel like enough. Afterwards, I felt ashamed and confused, and inevitably, fall into yet another consuming project.

I promise myself to not let this 'happen' again – instead, to put more effort into deciding what to buy and having some sort of 'throw as I go routine,' in other words, do things properly.

Dear Reader, may I invite you alongside me to view this experience through a lens of compassion.

Let's unpack this. A 'reset' feels necessary when I have spent ages hyper-focusing on a project. Routine falls apart around me, and the build-up begins – of paperwork, clothes, out-of-date food. When overwhelm strikes, I try outrunning the discomfort of it with activity. And it will happen again when I finish writing this book.

I can now feel compassion that for so long, I have berated myself for this pattern, even if it results in something meaningful getting done. My living space is small and busy with patterns and textures, so it looks 'extra messy' very quickly.

The experience of emerging from hyperfocus, leaving a beloved project behind, makes me feel bereft. And transitioning back to everyday tasks as well as from one mind state to another, is a combination that sends me into overwhelm. The need for instant simplicity is strong. Lately, I try to be kinder and remind myself that I am one person, and as such, can do only one thing at a time. Even though my brain finds this idea agony of a kind.

It's been super helpful to understand the universe's tendency towards entropy. To realise that a living space will naturally fall into disarray unless I spend most of my time maintaining it. Sod that!!

I work on finding self-compassion around

how I never see overwhelm rising like a tidal wave and hope, one day, to willingly yield to the understanding that my ADHD neurology needs to feel pressure enough to spark motivation, and that 'maintaining' isn't really an option for me. I'm trying to trust this process.

Problem? What Problem?

'There is no greater disability in society than the inability to see a person more.' – Robert N. Hensel.

2018

Recently, my person-centred counselling reading brought up an interesting question. If someone with a 'problem' is placed in an environment where they are understood, accepted and loved, how much of a 'problem' is there? How far is a 'problem' identified because of the way their difference is responded to within an environment.

Dear Reader, may I invite you alongside me to view this through a lens of compassion.

In the light of knowing I have ADHD neurology, when I ask myself this question, the answer becomes less about my deficit and more about the assumptions around ADHD in society.

My self-compassion about being a victim of such assumptions is mixed with the hope that they will quickly change. Maybe, if we can all raise awareness in some way, we will go on to feel that we have contributed to alleviating the struggles of all neurodivergent people, one voice at a time.

And Then I'm Gone

'Each spine was an encapsulated memory. Each book represented hours, days of pleasure, of immersion into words.' – Audrey Niffenegger.

2018

With kind, genuine interest while on a recent bookshop visit, my girlfriend asks me what I'm looking for. I can't be asked this question, as it feels immense, and I can't answer it. About to enter my 'process,' I give my practised, calm voiced reply that 'I'm not looking for, I'm looking at.' It's my way of steering her away. I ask her to please go off somewhere and come back later. She is used to this. We agree on a time, nod and synchronise watches.

I am looking for something, but my mind's eye is overwhelmed, and I'm staring without yet seeing, searching for the right pathway to begin the action of 'looking'. Most times, I just can't do it.

But in this instance, I make it safely to the

bookshelf. Mesmerised by the titles, each a little too captivating, there's a sensation of being pulled. I begin to swoon over each title which offers me the promise of a new, deep understanding. I can feel my usual strange anxiety starting – something between fear and excitement that has me fizzing inside and twitching. There's a slight light-headedness that makes me wonder whether I forgot breakfast.

And then I'm gone, opening books at random, reading sentences. I can't choose in a 'this one's better than that, because….' kind of way, only by a felt preference. And I trust myself with book purchases over other types of decisions but must take care to not suddenly have a 'felt preference' for them all.

It feels like five minutes before my friend is back. Tearing myself away is a mentally uncomfortable wrench, and I seem to have left my legs behind because, when I take the stairs, it's with the gait of an ungainly child.

Dear Reader, may I invite you alongside me to view this experience through a lens of compassion.

I hadn't realised that the way things happened in the bookshop, were much the same in other aspects of life. 'Felt preference' as a way of navigating life has always felt safer than trying to weigh things up in my head, and I can now begin to offer myself compassion around this, even tentatively embrace it.

Understanding the role that emotional memory plays in the life of a person with ADHD, that it's often equivalent to weighing up pros and cons offers us permission to move through life in ways that feel safer and more natural.

Wonderful or Torturous?

'It's the Way Things Are.' – Babe, Dick King-Smith.

I tell the counsellor I have recently hired for just a few sessions that I've read Marcus Aurelius' meditations and realise I don't think properly. I quote the stoic philosopher, 'You have power over your mind - not outside events. realise this, and you will find strength,'

'I do 'realise this,' I tell her, 'but my mind doesn't cooperate.' She narrows her eyes and tells me she needs more to understand completely. I invite her to join me at the bookshelf in Waterstones, explain the swooning and the promises, how I can't choose things in a 'normal' way, and how feeling 'torn away' when I'm concentrating makes me dizzy.

'I'm not sure if that sounds wonderful or torturous,' the counselor says. 'I could hear both.' She cocks her head questioningly, 'I'm wondering why you put yourself through it?'

I wonder whether she is asking me if I enjoy torture. How can I explain that I don't put myself through it? It happens.

I explain I feel sad and psychically bothered almost every day about my way of being. My way of thinking is like feelings thinking, not like 'thinking, thinking'. I am already uncomfortable, recognizing I'm worried about how much to say, as I begin sharing aloud, for the first time, one of my experiences of feeling 'different.'

The counsellor senses my discomfort and asks me to take my time. Disjoint-edly, I explain what not knowing how to make a decision properly means to me. I explain that 'properly' means comparing in your head. It's working through the features of two or more items. It's including and discarding with confidence. Purchasing items and making life decisions are particularly demanding. I tell her something in my head mixes everything up, and choosing becomes more guessing or gambling because I have to rely on a way of knowing I can't explain. I explain that perhaps this is different from actual gambling, which I suppose might have a more considered element or is inherently thrillingly risky. This, my 'decision-making process,' is like being forced to take a risk for want of a better way.

Dear Reader, may I invite you alongside me to view this childhood experience through a lens of compassion.

Later, I pondered my counsellor's earlier question, and realised that applied to supermarket shopping – I might have decided years ago that I just shouldn't. But despite the struggle, relating to survival, maybe there is something to be said for late-diagnosed ADHDers finding ways that, albeit quirky, worked. While, ADHD women of my generation could break their hearts with 'if only I'd known' (so tempting) so many are joyous with relief – because it's never too late to find self-acceptance.

Thank goodness, that as awareness around neurodivergence rises, the confusion around ADHD decreases.

Both wonderful and torturous as it is, I continue to frequent the realm of the bookshop.

The Article

'We cannot change what we are not aware of, and once we are aware, we cannot help but change.' – Sheryl Sandberg.

2019

My monthly therapy magazine lands on the mat, and I flick my eyes over the headings on the front page – strong, compelling subjects. I sit down that evening and start reading about adult ADHD. My son was diagnosed with ADHD, aged nineteen, and I wonder if I might gain insight into his world. I read that quite often that women with ADHD are misdiagnosed with depression. I didn't even know it was something girls had!

I read an anecdote, someone who found their diagnosis of ADHD to be the first step on their journey towards making sense of their lives. The article's author, a counsellor, writes that no one with ADHD walks the middle line, that for some people there is inattention and struggles with procrastination and for others, there is an internal motor that won't let them stop or relax. The types share many traits – including a low boredom threshold. I reflect with some relief that I don't get bored. I've always got ten things on the go, and anyway, I tend to get overwhelmed before I ever have a chance to get bored.

I read on but don't finish. It's not usual for me to lose my concentration mid-way. Place the magazine down, I feel an odd sense of urgency, yet need for a delay. I get a coffee and notice the dog is asking me for a walk. Back within fifteen minutes, the coffee is still warm. I remember I was doing something that felt very important. I search in the fuzzy inner detector way that I do, even attempting to retrace steps, but it's gone.

But something is beginning in me – a combined feeling of fear, hope and inner knowing. It grows gigantic in my chest, and I savour the flavour of hope. I begin a round of batch cooking, avoiding, convincing myself I'm too busy to sit down and read magazines. But eventually, I am drawn because a few days later, the article still sits open on the dining table. My curiosity and excitement eclipse my fear, and this time, the room falls away as I read.

ADHD Indicators:

People who speak incessantly

I think of how I feel when I interrupt people.

People who have feelings of stop-start underachievement patterns to college/university courses

It took me nine years on and off to complete my OU degree. Tick.

Disorganised life. A sense of overwhelm. Knowing what needs doing but being unable to do it – I think of all my undone things the almost physical feeling I get of, 'need to but can't'

(Conversely, don't I bash through some things with an unstoppable drive? Anyway, tick)

I read 'feelings of being driven by a motor, unable to stop and relax'

Vroom vroom, tick.

Job hopping

In a conversation with friends just last week, my announcement of having clocked up at least nine jobs before age twenty was my attempt at evidencing my strong work ethic. But I hadn't really wanted to share my experiences – all confusing. That I had felt an incongruence with my value system, one of quality over quantity, didn't escape me. Tick.

Risk-taking behaviour.

Daily feats of daring more than mortal risk-taking. Self-employment, performing in busy pubs, job changing, saying things I know are edgy, sending excessively assertive emails to schools...Tick.

Poor short-term memory.

Very. Tick.

Addictions

Do sugar, coffee and chocolate count? If so, legal, varied, ongoing.

Impulses

What are they? I'll have to look that up. I don't think of myself as impulsive.

I begin wondering whether how I think of myself has any bearing on how I actually am. Then:

> ADHD is about neurology and is hormone-connected, so it ramps for women in puberty and menopause.

Bingo. Might this explain why lately, I feel like I'm inhabiting my teenage self?

OK, This is What I Need to Think About

'A disorienting change pleases no one,
yet it builds self-made heroes.' – Auliq-Ice.

I take the online test - several. I read about overwhelm and meltdown. I read about someone living life in a way that seems too similar to my own. How can I relate to this? It feels intrusive. Strangers on Reddit understand more about me than I do! My most intimate struggles are exposed in anecdotes. For a while, I wanted to close my eyes and un-know.

I join ADDitude, the online magazine for people with ADHD, and became part of their supportive community. I write a blog, check out TotallyADD and appreciate Rick Green's honest, humourous, inform-ative approach and accessible Patreon community.

On Reddit, people share their mixed feelings about being 'textbook ADHD.' It resonates so much that I cry. I tentatively share my peculiar excitement with two of my closest friends and am amazed to find that they feel they share some of the same experiences. We thrash this out in our zoom chats, and realise why we are so close - it makes sense.

I decide that on the whole, this new understanding is mine to know and begin to journal. I start writing this book not knowing what the ending will be. Sometimes the intricacy of what I need to write to work things out seems ridiculous:

'OK, so this is what I need to think about; I might have an ADHD type of brain. If I have, then it answers all my little questions and my one big question all in one go. So, if this is the answer, then there was only ever one thing to know, and the way I am is because of it.'

Dear Reader, I invite you to view this experience through a lens of self-compassion.

The feeling of going into hyper-focus can be like my brain being swept out to sea while my body is left on the shore calling and calling until it's no longer heard. I feel compassion upon recognizing that without consciously permitting it, I can become peculiarly vulnerable in a public space.

Being an eighties child, 'feeling the burn' promised reward and

I believed that sending myself into the place I now know to be overwhelmed was some kind of 'muscle practice' for my brain - because, boy! It hurt!

In a world that demands efficient executive functions, a daily experience of overwhelm when trying to prioritise can feel exacerbated by choice and so, for the times I have experienced 'stuckness' and shame around my struggles with (supposedly simple) things, I am beginning to find self-compassion.

And for the part of myself that always longed to simplify life's every aspect – only to understand that to reduce choice this way requires a heft of decision-making that's too much for my brain, I feel sad.

I'm beginning to feel some compassion for my white-knuckle ride approach to 'sorting out,' during which my executive functioning challenged my ability to foresee that I might regret throwing something away! Setting alarms to break my hyperfocus or asking a friend to 'body double' with me is a good beginning.

Finding ADHD-friendly approaches is helping to create new opportunities around things I once believed impossible.

But I'll Still Have ADHD Next Year!

'To have faith is to trust yourself to the water. When you swim, you don't grab hold of the water because you will sink and drown if you do. Instead, you relax and float.' – Alan Watts.

2018

Before my diagnosis, I had booked myself onto a course to teach mindfulness to incorporate it into the therapy room as a 'tool' for my clients. This would mean going away for a week to become immersed in 'the moment' – several moments – to learn how I might appropriately share mindfulness with people to reduce stress. But with my work around my ADHD and self-compassion, I recognise that my neurology would be integral to how I would need to work as a facilitator. So I telephoned the college, thinking that perhaps I ought to cancel.

Despite my enthusiasm, it might be too much to offer something I struggle with. Maybe it would be unethical and suspect that what I think to be my mindfulness experience is really just the zoning out I now understand. I can't imagine ever being able to harness enough whatever-it-is to sit and be properly 'mindful of the moment.' I may not want to notice what's happening around me. Maybe I like zoning out! I suddenly realise that I am scared I will be bored on my cushion, in my head.

The lady on the telephone is lovely. I tell her I have recently been diagnosed with ADHD and that I'm unsure whether I should be doing the course – whether I can. I am processing this right now, so I ask her about my options. She kindly tells me we can postpone until later this year or next. I feel tearful, and something bubbles up in me, and I blurt out, 'But I'll still have ADHD next year! It won't go away! I'm always in a trait – I can't step outside them, this is it!' She is mortified, I can tell. And so am I, and begin to apologise.

She says, 'No, please. You have given me the necessary insight that having ADHD isn't an on-off thing.' She apologises, and I can tell she feels like she has just suggested to someone who has lost a leg that they can postpone their trampolining course until it grows back.

Dear Reader, I invite you to view this experience through a lens of self-compassion.

This first ADHD 'outing' was before I understood that I am not my traits. I feel self- compassion for the fear I felt that day, and before I understood that mindfulness is a fantastic way to get to know your 'present' self. That it's a refuge when my hyperfocus or hyperactivity has trawled me around for hours.

Shifting my awareness to tension in my face, neck, and shoulders, then to my breathing can bring me gently out of hyperfocus in a way that isn't jarring and help me slow my body in a way that slows my mind. Amazing!

The How of Things

'Life is made up of circles... Life is not a straight line... And sometimes we circle back to a past time. But we are not the same. We are changed forever.'
– Patricia MacLachlan.

2019

I began to feel confused about how to relate to myself. Are my feelings even my feelings? What part of me can I trust is uniquely me, not ADHD. My efforts to slow down that feel monumentally personal, do they belong to other people too? I notice I can't yet call it my ADHD like many people do, but I want to if it's as much a part of my way of being as I suspect. I'm worried that the moment I mention ADHD, there will be 'that look,' much like the one I pretend not to see.

And now, although I know that many people experience the same struggles, I feel more alone than ever.

In a vain attempt to feel OK, I do my usual rounds of daytime sleeping and decluttering – particularly of things I now recognise were bought on impulse. Now I know why it happens, I don't want to see 'the evidence.' I binge on boxsets and visit the online Ikea shop, whose products are like a promise that I might out-organise life as I know it.

All the while, these activities are monitored by my far away and wiser mind, remote and indistinct with a 'whu whaa woo whaa' parents in Peanuts feel. And although I can't tune in, I'm slowly becoming more present to my desperation.

Although painful, it feels important to get here. To this knowing – that nothing external will 'work', and that the rounds and rounds of my usual activities, my 'escaping,' just pull me further away from myself. The work I need to do will begin from within. Maybe, just maybe, that last round of those behaviours that significantly impact my health, time and bank balance is done.

But something feels important in my way of discerning importance - my textbook ADHD, non-logical gut-pulling way.

That I wouldn't change where my paths have led me – to here, to now, and perhaps this is important in itself? So often, the way I have approached things is where regret pops up. For example, promising a friend I will knit or paint for them suddenly turns it into a chore. But knowing, now, that my focus shifts to their expectation and reduces my ability to function, I might learn a new approach. Already I understand that, in contrast, a surprise gives me room to breathe. I may never finish, but I might. Hope is eco-fuel for my neurology whereas 'having to' is diesel.

When I think of how I've invested my love, time and energy only to find it is yet another 'learning curve.' I see now it's a learning circle, and I reflect that sometimes trusting my feelings and following my gut instinct would have led to better outcomes. But we live in a world that reveres our ability to 'think things through properly.'

Also, I recognise that the energy of youth, which felt like a given, coupled with the relentless hyperactivity of ADHD combined to create reflexive, not reflective days.

My new understanding of why I have always struggled with the how of things – the pace and intensity at which I negotiate my internal environment is a big thing.

But it doesn't follow that I know what to do with it!

I imagine my way will matter when I get to the end of my years, not my what, and I'm certain I won't celebrate how productive I have been. The moments that will matter will be those in which I am relaxed and present. This realisation is a bitter pill to swallow. Properly understanding all of this is beginning to matter hugely.

While I don't regret many whats of life, there's a question mark over some of the hows, and despite being fuelled by hyperactivity and driven by impulse, I am grateful that what I do is never dangerous. Or, is it?

I ponder on this. On the ways an ADHD size gap in my self-knowledge left me vulnerable in relationships, on years of not realising I needed to wind down to sleep or eat well. I ponder on the confusions, on trying to be who I thought I should be and the cruel self-speak that damaged my confidence, and conclude that there are different types of dangers.

Dear reader, may I invite you to view this experience through a lens of self-compassion

For at least a year, having ADHD was all I could talk about, think about and read about. This is usual for people diagnosed in mid-adulthood, and I feel compassion for everyone who begins realising the ways an ADHD neurology has impacted their life so far.

Self-compassion arises when I recall how left behind I felt upon finding that a whole, younger generation was already equipped with buzzwords and understanding about their ADHD struggles.

But their boldness and determination to 'live as they are' and to raise awareness won me over, made me join them. At their age, I had nothing to assert but confusion.

I moved, unsettled between regret (for what I believed life could have been), fear (of exposure before gaining a complete understanding), and relief (of having the answer to a lifetime of questions).

Then a new question arose: 'Where do I go from here?'

I wonder, despite having had a bit of fun with the idea of time travel, whether the fact that we can only start from where we are might be a blessing?

The quote about finding the grace to accept what we can't change has always resonated, and I can only imagine that for our neurodivergent forbears, this was a boggy mission.

Hopefully, for us, armed with new understandings about the reasons for our struggles, the ground upon which we stand to begin finding that grace feels much firmer.

Returning

'Time is only a kind of Space.' – HG Wells

1971

I am sitting on the grass in my childhood garden, aged around two.

I know the lady is here again, and I'm happy because I know she is just me – only taller, coming to enjoy the warm sun and whisper smiles in my ear. A bumblebee, a fuzzy ball, hums as it works from flower to flower. I notice a black dot crawling on my toe and the tiny tickle it brings. My breath is a burst that blends with the smells, colours, sounds, and sensations. This experience is of me, and I of it.

Dear Reader, I invite you to view this experience through a lens of self-compassion.

How fanciful it is, to suspend our disbelief and imagine we can visit our younger selves and offer them the promise of our strength and knowledge. Yes, as neurodivergent people a 'heads up' would have been very useful. Instead, somehow, we navigated our confusion and reached adulthood.

We might think of that 'somehow' as the sum total of the wealth of our resourcefulness to date, and testimony to our resilience.

Whisper Her a Future

'You know, if you hang around this earth long enough, you really see how things come full circle.' – Patti Davis.

Present Day

I sit beside my younger self and learn. Watch her wonder and know it was once mine, that it is still inside me, touching my dreams and infusing my hopes with sparkles. I whisper to her a future, the depth and breadth of all that one's inner world of ways can offer to a person with ADHD, and promise that on a later journey, a loop in time will bring her to revisit this moment as memory.

Now working with people with their mid-life diagnosis of ADHD, when I hear confusion in my therapy room, pain and a familiar gap in self-understanding, it is a privilege to meet my client 'where they are' and to walk beside them on their journey home to themselves.

Thank you, Dear Reader, for your

company. Keeping you in mind, by my side and in my heart has made writing this book possible.

Acknowledgments

With my heartfelt thanks to...

My lovely husband, Martin, who shares my passion for raising awareness about neurodivergence, and whose smiles light my days.

Danny, Tommy and Anna, my fantastic adult children, whose humour keeps me going.

Jess, and Stacie, my daughters-in-law, who I admire for being true to themselves.

My new adult step-children, Dale, Chloe and her partner Dan, for welcoming me to their family.

Auntie Julie, for encouraging me and advising on book structure.

'Angels' Gill and Suzanne, my dear friends and fellow counsellors, for your encouragement.

Monie, Di, Janice, Frida, Liz, Di, Catherine, Sue and Tabitha, all for your wonderful friendship and understanding.

Luke Smitherd, Author, whose fantastic stories reignited my writing journey.

All my hardworking clients whose resources amaze me, and my supervisor, Gillian, for her ongoing wisdom.

Catherine and the team at ADHDAware, Brighton, for guiding me as a volunteer.

Author and psychotherapist Sari Solden, for her generous review of Talking to a Pie, and for her amazing books for women with ADHD.

Dr Kristin Neff whose Self-Compassion work inspires me.

Mindfulness Now for their online MBSR training during Covid.

Lorraine and Peter, tutors on my counselling journey, for their gentle patience.

Arkbound's Bridget, my fabulous editor, for her energy and professionalism and Jennifer for generously giving her time to support production.

Everyone who expressed their belief in *Talking to a Pie about Walking the Dog* through crowdfunding – you got the ball rolling!

About the Author

Katy Fraser, BSc, Dip.Couns (MBACP)

Having been diagnosed with ADHD in her early fifties, Katy candidly and humorously reflects on and reexamines her often messy life. Providing a beacon of hope, Katy dismantles the stigma of the diagnosis, helping ADHDers feel profoundly understood. Katy enjoys time with her family, friends and dogs and is a psychotherapeutic counsellor now working with neurodivergent adults as her specialism.

Contact Katy Fraser at:
katyfraserauthor@gmail.com
https://www.katyfraser.com

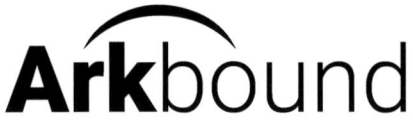

Writing · Publishing · Diversity · Inclusion

Our unyielding mission is to open up the
world of literature, journalism and publishing
to everyone through delivering mentoring,
workshops, events and sponsorship. We
believe that empowering people through
writing is a way towards building a stronger,
fairer and more enlightened society.

Building Futures. Bridging Divides.